PUBLIC HEALTH IN THE 21ST CENTURY

THE EVOLUTION OF HEALTH LITERACY

EMPOWERING PATIENTS THROUGH IMPROVED EDUCATION

PUBLIC HEALTH IN THE 21ST CENTURY

Additional books in this series can be found on Nova's website under the Series tab.

Additional e-books in this series can be found on Nova's website under the eBooks tab.

PUBLIC HEALTH IN THE 21ST CENTURY

THE EVOLUTION OF HEALTH LITERACY

EMPOWERING PATIENTS THROUGH IMPROVED EDUCATION

NITIN AGARWAL
DAVID R. HANSBERRY
AND
ARPAN V. PRABHU
EDITORS

nova science publishers
New York

Library of Congress Cataloging-in-Publication Data

ISBN: 978-1-53610-602-2

Library of Congress Control Number: 2016959466

Published by Nova Science Publishers, Inc. † New York

We dedicate this book to our patients, striving to advance and improve the field of health literacy. We are grateful that our patients entrust us with the opportunity learn and practice our trade. We would like to thank the Beckwith Institute as well for its commitment to our endeavors.

Nitin Agarwal, M.D.
David R. Hansberry, M.D., Ph.D.
Arpan V. Prabhu

CONTENTS

FOREWORD

What is health literacy? While many people equate health literacy with overall literacy, they are quite distinct. While literacy is the level to which an individual can read and write, the United States Department of Health and Human Services defines health literacy as: "the degree to which individuals have the capacity to obtain, process, and understand basic health information and services needed to make appropriate health decisions."

Almost every individual has been in a situation in which he or she doesn't understand what a physician is saying, but yet we do not speak up. How can we empower patients to feel comfortable asking questions, and equip physicians with the tools to support their patients and help them heal?

This book will provide physicians with an introduction to and history of health literacy in the United States. It uncovers the truth behind the comprehension levels of many of the printed health materials that patients are currently given. Each chapter of this book provides relatable and applicable learning that will ultimately and positively affect the level of your patients' understanding of their health.

- Learn how to develop text that your patients will easily understand, and how to gauge the readability of your current health materials.
- Become enlightened on how the Internet has changed the ways that patients receive health information.
- Embrace methods for assessing on line materials to better identify those that are appropriate for your patients.

On behalf of The Beckwith Institute, we are pleased to introduce this book, ***The Evolution of Health Literacy: Empowering Patients Through Improved Education***. We believe this book will change the way health care providers communicate with and educate their patients.

G. Nicholas Beckwith
Chairman, UPMC Board of Directors
Co-Founder, The Beckwith Institute
Board Chair, Clinical Transformation Program, The Beckwith Institute

Dotty Beckwith
Co-Founder, The Beckwith Institute
Board Chair, Frontline Innovation Program, The Beckwith Institute

PREFACE

Physicians have long pledged to adhere to four basic moral principles, a concise framework for the larger field of medical ethics. As is commonly known, those values consist of autonomy, beneficence, non-maleficence, and justice. However, in order to advocate for these principles for patients, medical professionals must first ensure patients have appropriate medical resources from which to glean information. This text serves to underscore this concept and advance the field of patient education.

In: The Evolution of Health Literacy
Editors: N. Agarwal et al.
ISBN: 978-1-53610-602-2

Chapter 1

Overview and History of Health Literacy in the United States and the Epidemiology of Low Health Literacy in Healthcare

Raghav Gupta[1], Christopher J. Kim[2], Christoph J. Griessenauer, MD[1], Ajith J. Thomas, MD[1], and Christopher S. Ogilvy, MD[1]

[1]Division of Neurosurgery, Beth Israel Deaconess Medical Center, Harvard Medical School, Boston, Massachusetts, US
[2]Rutgers New Jersey Medical School, Newark, New Jersey, US

Abstract

Health literacy has been touted as an important predictor of health care status in the United States. However its definition has rapidly evolved given the introduction of different media for the transmission of health-related information and an expanding base of medical knowledge. While a number of tools exist for evaluating one's health literacy level, the widespread adoption and accuracy of these methods, remains poorly understood. In the US alone millions are believed to be affected by low health literacy, rendering these patients incapable of making informed decisions within the clinical setting. Given the well-documented impact that low health literacy can have on one's health and ability to make use of public health care facilities, an understanding of the components of literacy and health literacy is prudent. The epidemiological determinants of health literacy, its origins, and its effects are reviewed.

1. Introduction

Given the increasing amount of health education materials disseminated via the Internet, social media, and print, the accountability rests on patients to decipher the plethora of information available. Accordingly the term 'health literacy' has been described as a new and evolving research discipline within clinical medicine and public health [1]. This chapter attempts to define health literacy within the broader framework of 'literacy' and provides an extensive overview of the history of the concept over the past two centuries. This chapter also discusses the potential impacts of low health literacy in healthcare and the epidemiological determinants of low health literacy.

2. Overview of the History of Health Literacy in the United States

2.1. Overview of Literacy in the United States

The National Literacy Act of 1991, introduced by Congress in an attempt to enhance the literacy skills of adults, defined literacy as: an "individual's ability to read, write, speak in English, compute and solve problems at a level of proficiency necessary to function on the job and in society, to achieve one's goals, and to develop one's knowledge and potential" [2].

Over time, however, the operational definition for 'literacy' in the United States has evolved dramatically. Berkman et al. posited that around the time of the American Civil War, literacy was measured by an individual's ability to sign a legal document with his or her name, rather than by writing an 'X.' This definition evolved and between the late 19th century and early 20th century, the United States Census Bureau began asking individuals if they could read or write in any language in an attempt to more accurately measure literacy across the American population. It was determined that nearly 20% of the population was illiterate in the late 19th century. By 1979, however, this number had decreased to only 0.6% of the population. Although the legitimacy of the early measures of literacy in the American population is dubious, a decrease in the number of illiterate Americans is clearly suggested [2].

Throughout the 20th century, increasingly complex definitions and measurements of literacy began to arise as both the military and civilian sectors of the work force were required to determine the necessary skills needed for a prospective hire to function on the job. As a result, the term "functional literacy" was coined. Throughout the twentieth century, literacy was measured relative to increasing levels of educational achievement and the ever-changing demands of the expanding labor force. In the 1950's, functional literacy was defined by the US Census Bureau as having a sixth grade education at the minimum; this standard would later be raised to a minimum of an eighth grade education [2]. This standard has again been raised today: Snow et al. argues that a postsecondary education or training is required to be considered 'competitive' in the labor force [3, 4].

Despite the decrease in the number of illiterate citizens within the late twentieth century reported by Berkman, Davis, and McCormack, low literacy remains a problem in the United States even today [2]. In 1993, the National Adult Literacy Survey (NALS) reported that 90 million Americans scored in the lowest two levels out of a possible five-level scale of literacy. These 90 million Americans were deemed functionally illiterate and had difficulty integrating information obtained from complex texts or documents and performing calculations that required two or more sequential operations [5].

In the 1980s, leading researchers Carroll and Chall released the publication, "Toward a Literate Society," which also found that while illiteracy levels continued to decline, many Americans still suffered from severe and significant deficits in reading and comprehension [6]. A subsequent National Academy of Education report extolled the importance of developing an accurate, national measure of literacy prior to the implementation of any future interventional programs addressing literacy [2].

A number of indices were formed thereafter to measure levels of functional literacy within the American population. In 1985, the US Department of Education introduced the National Assessment of Educational Progress (NAEP), which was designed for use in adults between 21 and 25 years of age. In 1990, the US Department of Labor released an assessment and questionnaire collectively titled the, 'Literacy Proficiencies of Job Seekers' to better understand how well working-citizens were able to understand various forms of text. In 1993, the Department of Education introduced the National Adult Literacy Survey, which aimed to assess adult literacy throughout the entire US population. Furthermore, in 2003, the Department of Education introduced the National Assessment of Adult Literacy (NAAL) as a tool to measure the proportion of adults with "below basic skills" who required further education. The NAAL held significance to researchers of health literacy as it was "the first large scale national literacy assessment that contained a component specifically designed to measure health literacy in all US adults" [2].

2.2. Emergence of Health Literacy

It is clear that education on basic health and hygiene has been a key component of promoting better lifestyles and preventing the spread of disease throughout contemporary medical history. According to Nutbeam et al., developed nations utilized health education as a means of promoting general health as well as preventing communicable diseases from ravaging entire populations, particularly in the 1960s and 1970s, such as the 1964 Surgeon General's report on smoking. However, it became increasingly evident that campaigns were ineffective when they were based upon the distribution of large quantities of information, without taking into account the socioeconomic status of the population to which they were targeted. The majority of the health promotion programs in the 1970s, as it turned out, were only effective in assisting the previously educated and economically advantaged populations [7, 9].

In the late 20th century, the emphasis of public health initiatives had shifted from addressing the devastating living and working conditions witnessed during the industrial revolution to modifying individual health behaviors. Public health scholars were taking a particular interest in studies that investigated the usefulness of social, economic, and environmental conditions and policies as determinants of health [7]. Indeed, the Ottawa Charter for Health Promotion, held in 1986, reflected this interest in its call for commitment to health promotion [8]. Here, good health was described as being not only a lifestyle choice, but also a state of well being that ideally should be achieved by all. Nutbeam et al. purport that such an emphasis in modifying individual health behaviors led to the development or rise of health literacy, which quantified an individual's ability to access, understand, and use the information provided to them to improve and maintain good health [9].

A wealth of research and work in the field of health literacy has been contributed [1, 2, 5, 10-14], ranging broadly from studies offering improved definitions of health literacy, evaluating potential interventions to improve low levels of health literacy, to examining health literacy as a risk factor for health issues. Policymakers and scientists in the 1990's focused on defining health literacy by initially measuring its prevalence and examining its associations and epidemiology [1]. The importance of health literacy was summarized in the Institute of Medicine's 2004 report *Health Literacy: A Prescription to End Confusion*, which stated, "efforts to improve quality, reduce costs, and reduce disparities in healthcare cannot succeed without simultaneous improvements in health literacy" [1, 15].

2.3. Health Literacy: An Evolving Definition

The American Medical Association's Ad Hoc Committee on Health Literacy noted that the term 'health literacy' had existed in the health literature for at least 30 years without a clear working definition [9]. Ironically, the definition of health literacy is still evolving, as it is a relatively new construct. The definition of health literacy, as a result, has been inconsistently applied across several studies [12]. Guzys et al. states that this may be due to the concept of health literacy "having a cluster of attributes, rather than a strict set of attributes that are subject to change as they are prioritized differently by different groups of people." Indeed, one review indicates that from 1999 to 2010, seventeen health literacy-related articles were published that contained nearly thirteen different definitions of health literacy [2].

Berkman et al. noted that early definitions of health literacy focused only "on the ability to apply basic reading and mathematical (numeracy) skills in a health care context." However, an alternative and widely cited definition focuses on the "goal of being health literate" or "having the capacity to obtain, process, and understand medical information in a health related context," rather than simply applying previously learned skills from one situation to another [2].

A definition of health literacy, included in a 2004 Institute of Medicine report, has also been widely cited throughout the medical literature. The report defines health literacy as "the degree to which individuals have the capacity to obtain, process, and understand basic health information and services needed to make appropriate health decisions" [2, 15].

2.4. Assessment of Health Literacy

A few methods for assessing health literacy have been reported. Commonly utilized methods include the Rapid Estimate of Adult Literacy in

Medicine (REALM) and the Test of Functional Health Literacy in Adults (TOFHLA). However, REALM and TOFHLA both place an emphasis on reading-related skills and thus are not considered adequate assessments of skills required in a healthcare setting [2].

REALM, developed in the early 1990's, tests reading ability through word recognition and pronunciation. Scores range from 0 to 66: a patient who scores between 0 and 18 likely will not be able to read most low literacy materials, or materials aimed at low literacy audiences, and will require supplementary information. A patient who scores between 19 and 44 will require low literacy materials and may not be able to read prescription labels. A patient who scores between 45 and 60 will likely struggle with average patient education materials. A score between 61 and 66 indicates adequate health literacy [16].

TOFHLA, developed in the mid 1990's, measures the ability to read and understand prose passages. Scores range from 0 to 100, where a score between 0 and 59 indicates inadequate health literacy; a score between 60 and 74 indicates marginal health literacy; and a score between 75 and 100 indicates adequate health literacy [17].

2.5. Health Literacy: An Area for Improvement

According to a 2011 report published in the *Annals of Internal* Medicine, approximately 80 million US adults are believed to have limited or insufficient health literacy [18]. Such a deficiency likely puts these adults at risk for poorer health outcomes. Indeed, poor health literacy has been attributed to an increased risk of mortality (nearly two-fold increase), increased hospitalization and healthcare utilization [19-21], and poorer overall health, all of which seem to be particularly pertinent in the elderly population [18, 22, 23].

As a result, health literacy is one of the four key priorities of public health in the United States, and multiple agencies and organizations including the Department of Health and Human Services, the Joint Commission on the Accreditation of Healthcare Organizations, and the American Medical Association, have listed health literacy as a crucial patient safety and quality of care issue [19, 24].

However, despite health literacy being listed as a key priority for many healthcare-related organizations and agencies, limited awareness of the importance of health literacy has been cited as an area of concern. A 2013 article authored by Pleasant et al. suggested that health literacy is garnering increased attention, as indicated by the rapid growth in the number of healthliteracy related publications. However, it is likely that far more people are unaware of the notion than are aware of it. The study reported on the results of a global survey of 300 individuals working in the field of health literacy. The responses suggested that while the respondents strongly agreed that health literacy was an issue that needed to be addressed, nearly half felt it was one that evaded public attention and understanding [13].

The prevalence of low health literacy in the United States has led to calls for interventions to address the issue [1, 10, 21, 25]. Given the number of working definitions for the term 'health literacy,' it becomes difficult for researchers to adequately determine whether certain measures will have measurable effects. In addition, the limitations of current methods in measuring and assessing health literacy have been cited as an area of concern. Guzys et al. report that while a number of tools exist for assessing health literacy in healthcare settings, these assess word recognition, reading comprehension, and functional health literacy through 'informal measures.' Such informal measures include assessing patient health literacy by frequency of missed appointments or submissions of incomplete medical forms [12]. These data are therefore highly subjective in nature, limiting their utility.

3. Epidemiology of Low Health Literacy in Healthcare

Various studies have examined epidemiological factors associated with low health literacy. Understanding the racial and socioeconomic determinants of health literacy is essential to developing robust interventions capable of successfully targeting various demographic groups. For example, certain ethnic groups (i.e., African Americans) have been associated with low levels of health literacy [32, 35-39]. Having a low level of education has also been cited as being a strong risk factor for health illiteracy [5, 17, 20, 23, 24, 40-49]. Even age-dependent differences in health literacy skills have been reported [27-34]. How are the three factors related? Can we predict which groups of citizens will likely benefit the most from systemic changes?

3.1. Education and Low Health Literacy

Many studies have reported low education levels and attainment as predictors of inadequate or impaired health literacy. However, studies have conflicted over the strength of the correlation between the two. Martin et al. found lower educational attainment to be the strongest predictor of inadequate health literacy among nine variables studied [41], which is consistent with other reports [40, 47]. However, Baker et al. reported limited association between educational attainment and literacy [17], and Taha et al. determined that educational levels were not significant predictors of literacy as measured by TOFHLA and the Subjective Numeracy Scale (SNS), which assesses numeracy as a predictor of literacy level [48]. These effects are often hard to study given the number of confounding variables (i.e., age and race) that are present. It is important to note that correlation does not imply causation in these cases. In the future, such studies have to control for various social and economic determinants that may cloud the relationship between education status and health literacy.

3.2. Racial Differences and Low Health Literacy

Racial disparities have also been cited as strong predictors of inadequate health literacy. Chaudhry et al. found that being African American was strongly associated with worse health literacy, suggesting that important challenges exist in addressing health disparities in black patients [43]. Morrow et al. also found that race was a significant predictor of low literacy, along with gender, education, and cognitive variables [45]. Martin et al. reported that race and ethnicity were strongly associated with health literacy, with Blacks and Hispanics having significantly lower health literacy than non-Hispanic whites [41]. Several additional studies have focused on the prevalence of low health literacy in African Americans societies [43, 47, 49, 50]. Again, such types of analyses are complex, given the number of variables present at one time. Could the level of education within these societies have been inherently lower? Is it possible that access to education was limited in the first place? These are the questions that healthcare policymakers and clinicians are tasked with answering in the upcoming decades.

3.3. Age and Impairments in Health Literacy

Age has inconsistently been cited as a predictor of inadequate health literacy. Baker et al. wrote that functional health literacy was evidently lower in older age groups [23, 27]. Kobayashi et al. proposed that health literacy skills exhibited differential patterns of age-related change, which was attributed to cognitive aging [28]. Bostock and Steptoe agreed, suggesting that increasing age and decline in general cognitive abilities are tied hand-in-hand and are indicators of poor health literacy [29]. However, Shea et al. found that increasing age was a predictor of lower scores on the REALM examination when stratification by education level was not performed [47]. This suggests that age alone may not be an adequate predictor of health literacy. Other factors associated with increasing age should be considered, as discussed previously.

4. Impact of Low Health Literacy on Health

Low health literacy has been associated with a number of health impairments, including poorer general health [2, 5, 9, 17, 21, 24, 52], increased risk of hospital admission [53], increased mortality in the elderly [22, 23, 44, 54], increased rates of obesity [55], increased use of emergent health services [18], and poorer health amongst HIV patients [46, 49, 52].

4.1. Risk of Hospital Admission

Inadequate health literacy has been associated with an increased risk of hospital admission [53]. Baker et al. found that, after adjusting for age, gender, race, self-reported health, socioeconomic status, and health insurance coverage, health illiterate patients were at significantly higher risk of hospital admission than literate patients. Illiterate patients were found to be older, possess Medicare, report poorer health, lack a car, and have lower levels of educational attainment [53]. Illiterate patients were also more likely to have a wide array of problems in communicating with healthcare providers, were less likely to exercise, were prone to misusing prescription medications, and were more likely to practice adverse health behaviors (including smoking, alcohol, or drug use).

4.2. Obesity

Individuals with inadequate health literacy were found to have difficulty adhering to a healthy lifestyle and maintaining a healthy weight and diet. A possible link between inadequate health literacy and abnormal body mass index (BMI) was found in African American women who had difficulty accessing and understanding nutritional information [55].

4.3. Use of Health Services

Inadequate health literacy has been associated with increased use of emergency care services and healthcare services, a lower probability of utilizing preventative health services like mammograms and immunizations, and an inability to appropriately take medications and adhere to a prescribed treatment regimen [18].

4.4. Management of HIV/AIDS Patients

Limited or inadequate health literacy in HIV/AIDS patients has been associated with increased risk of medication nonadherence [46, 49], lower CD4 cell counts, a greater number of hospitalizations, and poorer self-reported health [52].

5. Health Literacy and the Burden to the Healthcare System

Of significant interest is the impact and burden of inadequate health literacy on the healthcare system. According to the National Institutes of Health, health illiteracy costs the United States healthcare system between $106-$236 billion annually. They go on to further implicate limited patient health literacy and understanding as causes of increasing healthcare expenditures, decreased access to health care, and decreased quality of care [56]. Rasu et al. suggested that health literacy is inversely correlated with healthcare utilization and expenditure and found that health illiterate patients spend more on prescription drugs and incur significantly higher medical expenses than individuals with adequate health literacy [19]. Public health interventions and improvements addressing inadequate health literacy in the American population may help improve the general health of the American public and simultaneously address the exponentially rising health care costs in the United States.

REFERENCES

[1] Parker R, Ratzan SC. Health Literacy: A Second Decade of Distinction for Americans. *J. Health Commun.* 2010;15:20-33. doi:10.1080 /10810730.2010.501094.

[2] Berkman ND, Davis TC, McCormack L. Health Literacy: What Is It? *J. Health Commun.* 2010;15(52):9-19. doi:10.1080/10810730.2010. 499985.

[3] Snow C, Biancarosa G. *Adolescent Literacy and the Achievement Gap: What Do We Know and Where Do We Go from Here?* New York; 2003.

[4] Spellings MA. *Test of Leadership: Charting the Future of US Higher Education*. Jessup, MD; 2006.

[5] Dewalt D a, Berkman ND, Sheridan S, Lohr KN, Pignone MP. Literacy and health outcomes: a systematic review of the literature. *J. Gen. Intern. Med.* 2004;19:1228-1239. doi:10.1111/j.1525-1497.2004. 40153.x.

[6] Carroll, J. B., & Chall, J. S. (1975). Toward a literate society. New York: McGraw-Hill.

[7] Nutbeam D. The evolving concept of health literacy. *Soc. Sci. Med.* 2008;67(12):2072-2078. doi:10.1016/j.socscimed.2008.09.050.

[8] WHO. The Ottawa Charter for Health Promotion. In: Ottawa; 1986.

[9] Nutbeam D. Health literacy as a public health goal: a challenge for contemporary health education and communication strategies into the 21st century. *Health Promot. Int.* 2000; 15(3):259-267. doi:10.1093 /heapro/15.3.259.

[10] Ratzan SC. Health literacy: communication for the public good. *Health Promot. Int.* 2001;16(2):207-214. doi:10.1093/heapro/16.2.207.

[11] Kickbusch I, Maag D. Health literacy. *Int. Encycl. Public Heal.* 2008: 204-211. doi:10. 1080/00981389.2011.585703.

[12] Guzys D, Kenny A, Dickson-Swift V, Threlkeld G. A critical review of population health literacy assessment. *BMC Public Health.* 2015;15 (215):1-7. doi:10.1186/s 12889-015-1551-6.

[13] Pleasant A, Cabe J, Patel K, Cosenza J, Carmona R. Health Literacy Research and Practice: A Needed Paradigm Shift. *Health Commun.* 2015;30(12):1176-1180. doi:10. 1080/10410236.2015.1037426.

[14] Smith CA, Keselman A. Meeting Healthcare needs.pdf. In: *Meeting Health Information Needs Outside of Healthcare - Opportunities and Challenges*. Waltham, MA: Chandos Publishing; 2015:19-34.

[15] Nielsen-Bohlman L, Panzer A, Kindig DA. *Health Literacy: A Prescription to End Confusion*. Washington, D.C.; 2004.

[16] Davis T, Crouch M, Long S. *Rapid Estimate of Adult Literacy in Medicine (REALM) - Examiner's Instruction Sheet*. Red Lake, MN; 1998.

[17] Baker DW, Parker RM, Williams M V, Clark WS, Nurss J. The relationship of patient reading ability to self-reported health and use of health services. *Am. J. Public Health.* 1997;87(6):1027-1030. doi:10.2105/AJPH.87.6.1027.

[18] Berkman ND, Sheridan SL, Donahue KE, Halpern DJ, Crotty K. Low Health Literacy and Health Outcomes : An Updated Systematic Review. *Ann. Intern. Med.* 2011;155(2): 97-107.

[19] Rasu RS, Bawa WA, Suminski R, Snella K, Warady B. Health Literacy Impact on National Healthcare Utilization and Expenditure. *Int. J. Heal Policy Manag*. 2015;4 (11):747-755. doi:10.15171/ijhpm.2015.151.

[20] Ownby RL, Acevedo A, Waldrop-Valverde D, Jacobs RJ, Caballero J. Abilities, skills and knowledge in measures of health literacy. *Patient Educ. Couns*. 2014;95(2):211-217. doi:10.1016/j.pec.2014.02.002.

[21] Pignone M, DeWalt DA, Sheridan S, Berkman N, Lohr KN. Interventions to Improve Health Outcomes for Patients with Low Literacy. *J. Gen. Intern. Med.* 2005;20:185-192. doi:10.1111/j.1525-1497.2005.40208.x.

[22] Sudore RL, Yaffe K, Satterfield S et al. Limited literacy and mortality in the elderly: The health, aging, and body composition study. *J. Gen. Intern. Med*. 2006;21:806-812. doi:10.1111/j.1525-1497.2006.00539.x.

[23] Baker DW, Wolf MS, Feinglass J, Thompson JA, Gazmararian JA, Huang J. Health Literacy, Cognitive Abilities, and Mortality Among Elderly Persons. *J. Gen. Intern. Med.* 2008;23(6):723-726. doi:10.1007 /s11606-008-0566-4.

[24] Clement S, Ibrahim S, Crichton N, Wolf M, Rowlands G. Complex interventions to improve the health of people with limited literacy: A systematic review. *Patient Educ. Couns.* 2009;75:340-351. doi:10.1016 /j.pec.2009.01.008.

[25] Sheridan SL, Halpern DJ, Viera AJ, Berkman ND, Donahue KE, Crotty K. Interventions for Individuals with Low Health Literacy: A Systematic Review. *J. Health Commun.* 2011;16:30-54. doi:10.1080/10810730.2011.604391.

[26] Serper M, Patzer RE, Curtis LM et al. Health Literacy, Cognitive Ability, and Functional Health Status among Older Adults. *Health Serv. Res*. 2014;49(4):1249-1267. doi:10.1111/1475-6773.12154.

[27] Baker DW, Gazmararian JA, Sudano J, Patterson M. The association between age and health literacy among elderly persons. *J. Gerontol. B Psychol. Sci. Soc. Sci.* 2000;55(6): S368-S374. http://www.ncbi.nlm.nih.gov/pubmed/11078114. Accessed March 1, 2016.

[28] Kobayashi LC, Smith SG, O'Conor R et al. The role of cognitive function in the relationship between age and health literacy: a cross-sectional analysis of older adults in Chicago, US. *BMJ Open.* 2015;5(4): e007222. doi:10.1136/bmjopen-2014-007222.

[29] Bostock S, Steptoe A. Association between low functional health literacy and mortality in older adults: longitudinal cohort study. *BMJ.* 2012;344:e1602. http://www.pubmed central.nih.gov/articlerender.fcgi ?artid=3307807&tool=pmcentrez&rendertype=abstract. Accessed February 29, 2016.

[30] Garcia-Retamero R, Galesic M, Gigerenzer G. Do icon arrays help reduce denominator neglect? *Med. Decis. Making.* 30(6):672-684. doi: 10.1177/0272989X10369000.

[31] Morrow D, Clark D, Tu W et al. Correlates of health literacy in patients with chronic heart failure. *Gerontologist.* 2006;46(5):669-676. http://www.ncbi.nlm.nih.gov/pub med/17050758. Accessed February 19, 2016.

[32] Martin LT, Ruder T, Escarce JJ et al. Developing predictive models of health literacy. *J. Gen. Intern. Med.* 2009;24(11):1211-1216. doi:10.1007/s11606-009-1105-7.

[33] Peterson PN, Shetterly SM, Clarke CL et al. Health literacy and outcomes among patients with heart failure. *JAMA*. 2011;305(16):1695-1701. doi:10.1001/jama.2011.51 2.

[34] Taha J, Sharit J, Czaja SJ. The impact of numeracy ability and technology skills on older adults' performance of health management tasks using a patient portal. *J. Appl. Gerontol.* 2014;33(4):416-436. doi: 10.1177/0733464812447283.

[35] Chaudhry SI, Herrin J, Phillips C et al. Racial disparities in health literacy and access to care among patients with heart failure. *J. Card. Fail.* 2011;17(2):122-127. doi:10. 1016/j.cardfail.2010.09.016.

[36] Osborn CY, Paasche-Orlow MK, Davis TC, Wolf MS. Health literacy: an overlooked factor in understanding HIV health disparities. *Am. J. Prev. Med.* 2007;33(5):374-378. doi:10.1016/j.amepre.2007.07.022.

[37] Patel PJ, Joel S, Rovena G et al. Testing the utility of the newest vital sign (NVS) health literacy assessment tool in older African-American patients. *Patient Educ. Couns.* 2011;85(3):505-507. doi:10.1016 /j.pec.2011.03.014.

[38] Shea JA, Beers BB, McDonald VJ, Quistberg DA, Ravenell KL, Asch DA. Assessing health literacy in African American and Caucasian adults: disparities in rapid estimate of adult literacy in medicine (REALM) scores. *Fam. Med.* 2004;36(8):575-581. http:// www.ncbi. nlm.nih.gov/pubmed/15343419. Accessed March 1, 2016.

[39] Waldrop-Valverde D, Osborn CY, Rodriguez A, Rothman RL, Kumar M, Jones DL. Numeracy skills explain racial differences in HIV medication management. *AIDS Behav.* 2010;14(4):799-806. doi:10.1007/s10461-009-9604-4.

[40] Peterson PN, Shetterly SM, Clarke CL et al. Health literacy and outcomes among patients with heart failure. *JAMA*. 2011;305(16):1695-1701. http://www.pubmedcentral. nih.gov/articlerender.fcgi?artid=4540335&tool=pmcentrez&rendertype=abstract. Accessed March 1, 2016.

[41] Martin LT, Ruder T, Escarce JJ et al. Developing predictive models of health literacy. *J. Gen. Intern. Med.* 2009;24(11):1211-1216. http://www.pubmedcentral.nih.gov/articlerender.fcgi?artid=2771237&tool=pmcentrez&rendertype=abstract. Accessed March 1, 2016.

[42] Kobayashi LC, Smith SG, O'Conor R et al. The role of cognitive function in the relationship between age and health literacy: a cross-sectional analysis of older adults in Chicago, US. *BMJ Open*. 2015;5(4): e007222. http://www.pubmedcentral.nih.gov/ articlerender.fcgi?artid=4410118&tool=pmcentrez&rendertype=abstract. Accessed February 24, 2016.

[43] Chaudhry SI, Herrin J, Phillips C et al. Racial disparities in health literacy and access to care among patients with heart failure. *J. Card. Fail.* 2011;17(2):122-127. http://www. pubmedcentral.nih.gov/ articlerender.fcgi?artid=3053061&tool=pmcentrez&rendertype=abstract. Accessed March 1, 2016.

[44] Bostock S, Steptoe A. Association between low functional health literacy and mortality in older adults: longitudinal cohort study. *BMJ.* 2012;344:e1602. http://www.pubmed central.nih.gov/articlerender. fcgi ?artid=3307807&tool=pmcentrez&rendertype=abstract. Accessed February 29, 2016.

[45] Morrow D, Clark D, Tu W et al. Correlates of health literacy in patients with chronic heart failure. *Gerontologist.* 2006;46(5):669-676. http://www.ncbi.nlm.nih.gov/pub med/17050758. Accessed February 19, 2016.

[46] Osborn CY, Paasche-Orlow MK, Davis TC, Wolf MS. Health literacy: an overlooked factor in understanding HIV health disparities. *Am. J. Prev. Med.* 2007;33(5):374-378. http://www.sciencedirect.com/science /article/pii/S0749379707004655. Accessed February 15, 2016.

[47] Shea JA, Beers BB, McDonald VJ, Quistberg DA, Ravenell KL, Asch DA. Assessing health literacy in African American and Caucasian adults: disparities in rapid estimate of adult literacy in medicine (REALM) scores. *Fam. Med.* 2004;36(8):575-581. http:// www.ncbi.nlm .nih.gov/pubmed/15343419. Accessed March 1, 2016.

[48] Taha J, Sharit J, Czaja SJ. The impact of numeracy ability and technology skills on older adults' performance of health management tasks using a patient portal. *J. Appl. Gerontol.* 2014;33(4):416-436. http://www.ncbi.nlm.nih.gov/pubmed/24781964. Accessed February 24, 2016.

[49] Waldrop-Valverde D, Osborn CY, Rodriguez A, Rothman RL, Kumar M, Jones DL. Numeracy skills explain racial differences in HIV medication management. *AIDS Behav.* 2010;14(4):799-806. http://www. pubmedcentral.nih.gov/articlerender.fcgi?artid =2891293&tool=pmcentrez&rendertype=abstract. Accessed March 1, 2016.

[50] Patel PJ, Joel S, Rovena G et al. Testing the utility of the newest vital sign (NVS) health literacy assessment tool in older African-American patients. *Patient Educ. Couns.* 2011;85(3):505-507. http://www.ncbi. nlm.nih.gov/pubmed/21514089. Accessed February 27, 2016.

[51] Nguyen TH, Park H, Han H-R et al. State of the science of health literacy measures: Validity implications for minority populations. *Patient Educ. Couns.* 2015;98:1492-1512. doi:10.1016/j.pec. 2015.07.013.

[52] Kalichman SC, Rompa D. Functional Health Literacy is Associated with Health Status and Health-Related Knowledge in People Living with HIV-AIDS. *J. Acquir. Immune Defic. Syndr.* 2000;25(4):337-344.
[53] Baker DW, Parker RM, Williams M V, Clark WS. Health Literacy and the Risk of Hospital Admission. *J. Gen. Intern. Med.* 1998;13:791-798. doi:10.1046/j.1525-1497. 1998.00242.x.
[54] Moser DK, Robinson S, Biddle MJ et al. Health Literacy Predicts Morbidity and Mortality in Rural Patients With Heart Failure. *J. Card. Fail.* 2015;21(8):612-618. doi: 10.1016/j.cardfail.2015.04.004.
[55] James DCS, Harville C, Efunbumi O, Martin MY. Health literacy issues surrounding weight management among African American women: a mixed methods study. *J. Hum. Nutr. Diet.* 2015;28 Suppl. 2:41-49. http://www.ncbi.nlm.nih.gov/pubmed/24890122. Accessed March 1, 2016.
[56] National Institues of Health: Clear communciation - health literacy. Available at: http:// www.nih.gov/clearcommunication/healthliteracy .htm. Accessed March 2, 2016.

In: The Evolution of Health Literacy
Editors: N. Agarwal et al.
ISBN: 978-1-53610-602-2

Chapter 2

PRINTED EDUCATION MATERIALS: ANALYSIS, TEXT DEVELOPMENT AND INTERVENTIONS

***Varun Ayyaswami*[1], *Anshum Sood*[1], *Rafey Feroze*[2] *and Logan Pyle, DO*[3]**
[1]University of Maryland School of Medicine, Baltimore MD, US
[2]University of Pittsburgh School of Medicine, Pittsburgh, PA, US
[3]Department of Neurology, University of Pittsburgh Medical Center, Erie, PA, US

ABSTRACT

Printed health materials are widely used in health education and literacy. While it is common for health professionals to verbally educate patients, there is a strong need to reinforce patient education through the use of printed health materials to ensure patient understanding of treatment instructions. Unfortunately, although 90 million Americans read below a seventh grade level, the vast majority of printed health materials for patient education and instruction are written at an 8th-12th grade reading level. In this commentary, we discuss the use of the Flesch-Kincaid Reading Ease test, Simple Measure of Gobbledygook (SMOG) Formula, and Suitability Assessment of Materials (SAM) Trial to assess reading level in printed health materials. We then discuss crucial factors one must consider in the construction of the text of printed materials including organization, word and sentence structure, and the appropriate use of medical jargon. Finally, we examine the use of tailored or individualized printed health education interventions. Ultimately, we conclude that the construction of printed materials is vital to patient health education and urge health providers to take care to construct materials that can be understood and appreciated by their patients.

INTRODUCTION

Printed health materials including brochures, pamphlets, articles, newsletters, flyers, leaflets, and other text or image-based documents are widely used in health education and literacy. Their distribution has helped mold the foundation of a wide variety of health education interventions. While it is common practice for health professionals to verbally educate patients, it is highly recommended that reading material be used in conjunction with verbal education to reinforce communicated material and positively impact patent understanding of health and disease [1]. Patients, especially those in elderly and anxious populations, often forget vital medical information verbally relayed by a doctor. Although patients are more likely to concentrate on diagnosis-related information, many cannot recall the detailed treatment instructions relayed by providers [2]. Thus, written materials are useful in reinforcing to patients the information that is presented verbally. Moreover, having accessible educational material, most frequently in print form, is considered to be the basis of consumer involvement in healthcare, such that patients can feel actively engaged in managing their own health [3]. Printed materials in the form of pamphlets have been shown to potentially improve knowledge, attitudes, and behavior related to health issues [4]. However, the effectiveness of printed material was shown to be strongly dependent on implementation factors. These include their use in specific patient subgroups as opposed to general public samples as well as their use as a standalone or combination intervention [4].

The purpose of this commentary is to examine the factors that can improve patient comprehension of the text of printed health materials in order to better patient health literacy as well as health outcomes. To accomplish this, we will begin with a thorough analysis of the average patients reading level and provide the tools most helpful in the assessment of the reading level of printed materials. Next, we examine the crucial factors that need to be considered during the construction of the text of printed health materials. Finally, we conclude with a section reviewing the effectiveness of several printed heath material interventions to personalize or 'tailor' printed health materials to individuals.

METHODS

Understanding and Assessing Reading Level in Printed Health Materials

Understanding Patient Reading Level

In designing and implementing effective printed health materials it is crucial to understand the audience for which it is used. More than half the adults in the United States may have trouble comprehending health information. In fact, up to 90 million people in the United States have reading comprehension ability below that of a seventh grade level [5]. Moreover, 36% of people have only basic or below basic healthy literacy skills as determined by the National Assessment of Adult Literacy using a scale set forth by the Institute of Medicine and Healthy People 2010 [6]. However, at present, most printed health material for patient education and instruction are written at an 8th-12th grade reading level [7]. Thus, even when accessible, patients have difficulty understanding health materials provided to them, greatly decreasing their effectiveness. Therefore, it is essential to create and distribute printed health material that is written between the 3rd to 7th grade reading level. There are many widely available tests to measure and assess the grade level of a written document as well as its readability. We recommend the use of the Flesch-Kincaid Reading Ease test, SMOG Formula, and SAM Trial to assess a reading level in printed health materials due to their widely documented use in published literature, ease of use in quickly and efficiently calculating scores, and/or their holistic approach in assessing readability.

Assessing Patient Reading Level: Flesch-Kincaid Reading Test

This test is made up of two subtests, the Flesch Kincaid Reading Ease test and the Flesch-Kincaid Grade Level Formula. The Reading Ease test grades text on a scale of 0-100, factoring in average sentence length (ASL) and average number of syllables per word (ASW). The formula for the Flesch Reading Ease score is: 206.835 – (1.015 x ASL) – (84.6 x ASW); the higher the score, the easier the document is to read [8]. The Flesch-Kincaid Grade Level test also uses average sentence length (ASL) and average number of syllables per word (ASW) to rate the text on a U.S school grade level using the formula (.39 x ASL) + (11.8 x ASW) – 15.59 [9]. A score of 5.0 on the Flesch-Kincaid Grade Level test indicates that a fifth grader is able to understand the document.

Assessing Patient Reading Level: SMOG Formula

The Statistical Measurement of Gobbledygook (SMOG) test was developed by McLaughlin and is used in assessing reading grade levels of documents with more than thirty sentences. It consists of grouping three sets of ten sentences, with one set from the beginning of the document, one from the middle, and one from the end. Within each group of ten sentences every word with three or more syllables is counted, including words that appear more than once. After adding up the total number of words counted, the SMOG Conversion Table is used to equate the number of words with more than three syllables to a grade level. In cases where the document has fewer than 30 sentences, a conversation factor is utilized to multiply the total number of words with three or more syllables prior to input into the SMOG Conversion Table [10].

Assessing Patient Reading Level: SAM Test

The Suitability Assessment of Materials (SAM) test was developed to not only examine the readability of material, but to also assess its usability for a low literate user. The tool takes into account six categories: content, literacy demand, graphics, layout/typography, learning stimulation/motivation, and cultural appropriateness. Twenty-two specific criteria are spread out among the six evaluation areas: four items are related to content (purpose evident, content about behavior, scope limited, and summary provided), five items on literacy (reading grade level, writing style with active voice, common words for vocabulary, content given, and road signs), five items on graphics (cover shows purpose, graphics, relevance of illustrations, lists or tables explained, and captions used), three items on layout and typography (layout factors, typography with font size and cues, and subheadings used), three items about learning stimulation and motivation (interaction used, behavior modeled, and motivation with self-efficacy), and two items about cultural appropriateness (cultural match and cultural image and examples). Each item is rated as 0 (not suitable), 1 (adequate), 2 (superior), or N/A (not applicable). The score is then summed across the different criteria, and a SAM percentage score is produced by dividing that sum by the total possible score (total items without N/A times two). A higher SAM percentage score is indicative of a more suitable quality of printed material [11]. Generally, 70-100 percent is considered to be superior material, 40-69% is adequate material; 0-39% is not suitable material [12].

Comparison of Flesch-Kincaid Reading Test, SMOG Formula, and SAM Test

Each of the different tests previously discussed have their own advantages and disadvantages. The Flesh-Kincaid Reading test is beneficial because it is already integrated into commonplace computer software such as the Microsoft Office suite and has a high correlation with other instruments [13]. However, one potential pitfall of the test is that the scores may underestimate level of difficulty in terms of the understandability of the text because the shortest word is not always the simplest or most familiar word [14]. Since the Flesh-Kincaid Reading Test solely takes into account average sentence length and average number of syllables per word, more qualitative and subjective features of texts such as frequency of particular verbiage cannot be taken into consideration. This same limitation also holds true for the SMOG Formula since it too takes into account the number of syllables used. However, the advantage of the SMOG Formula is that it is the most commonly used readability formula and has been adopted by the National Cancer Institute [13]. As compared to the other two tests, the SAM Test is unique in that it tests not only readability, but also usability and suitability because of the qualitative criteria included in the test such as cultural appropriateness and relevance of layout of text. However, one limitation of the SAM Test is that it requires training to be used effectively since an individual must manually score the text, which also makes it subject to inter-operator variability. We recommend that when analyzing printed health materials for reading level to select the most appropriate test based on the advantages and disadvantages discussed above.

ANALYSIS

Crucial Factors in the Construction of Printed Materials

Organization

As important as how health material is written, is how it is presented. The organization of written health education materials can directly affect how patients comprehend and respond to documents. Research has shown that making key messages easy to locate further increase the probability that they will be read and their message communicated [15]. As such, more important information should be presented earlier. In addition, the use of sub-headings is crucial in designing an effective written material because readers want to be able to quickly scan and pick up on pertinent information. Subheadings should include a summary of the take away points that section wishes to convey to readers. One effective technique is following up a subheading with key highlighted information in bullet form [16]. Since many readers will only briefly scan the document's headings, subheadings, and highlighted information [17], structuring the key points within this framework can help ensure readers pick up the main ideas of the document. Furthermore, the use of organizers such as headings before a text presentation allows readers to better frame their thoughts on an issue. Moreover, the technique helps to stimulate reader interest and can also make text look less daunting to read [18].

Research also shows that bullet points, as opposed to a paragraph of solid text, are better at gaining the reader's attention [19], helping readers follow procedures [20], and assisting readers to retain and understand information [21]. Another useful technique to present information is through the question and answer format. Placing relevant questions prior to texts helps to peak reader interest and group information into more manageable sections [22].

Short Words and Sentences

Short words and sentences should be used to enhance the readability of text. As mentioned earlier, many of the readability tests measure readability based on the length of words/sentences. Since a high percentage of the population has low literacy levels, it is important to write text in a way they can understand; short words are preferred and more easily understood in patient material [23]. For example, while many patients might not understand the word "immunizations," they do understand "shots" [24].

Additionally, written material should be created using commonly used words, keeping specific medical terminology to a minimum and introduced only on an as needed basis. People outside of the medical profession often have a hard enough time understanding healthcare information as it is. This is made even more difficult when specific medical jargon is used. For example, a patient may confuse "take with food" as "put in food" [24]. While medical jargon is important to have efficient communication between people in the healthcare field, it is not necessarily relatable to people outside the medical field. Simply put, if patients cannot understand what they are being told to do, they cannot follow through with a suggested action. Thus, written text needs to be able to translate medical terminology into commonly used words. See Table for examples of medical jargon and simpler alternatives.

Furthermore, people can respond to different words with similar meaning in markedly different ways based on a particular word's connotation. For example, a study conducted with senior citizens showed that while they responded negatively to the word "exercise," they had a much more positive response to the words "physical activity" [25]. It can be useful to utilize focus groups that represent the population of patients that the written health information is expected to reach and poll them on different word choice to help develop the most impactful documents. This will allow the identification of how population subgroups perceive words and appropriate adjustment of documents accordingly [25].

Explaining Necessary Medical Terms

There are cases in which simpler words cannot be substituted in place for some medical words/phrases. At times, substitution can actually make the text more complicated for readers. For example when talking about healthy eating and the importance of a low fat diet, it is difficult to avoid using the word "cholesterol" [24]. Thus, it then becomes important to further explain and breakdown such medical terms into concepts a lay reader can understand. For example, describing how cholesterol is a type of fat made by the body and found in animal products can help readers conceptualize and better understand the topic [24]. Similarly, sometimes a word can have a different connotation in a medical setting than in other lay settings. This is particularly apparent with the word "negative." In a casual setting, the word "negative" is usually associated with a deleterious connotation. However in a healthcare setting, having a "negative" test is, for the most part, a desired and beneficial outcome. Thus without much exposure to healthcare terminology, a patient might be misguided in their thinking and believe that having a "negative" test result is indicative of a poor prognosis [24].

Engaging Readers

It has been shown that reader interaction can increase reader interest and recall of information [23]. Examples of ways of engaging readers are to: include questions for the readers to respond to such as "how would you..." and leave space for readers to write in a response; including a brief quiz at the end of the subject matter to allow readers to test their understanding; ask readers to identify and underline key points in the material [26]. These methods permit for active learning on part of the reader, which can lead to better comprehension and understanding. Additionally, a study showed that readers reacted positively to being provided spaces in written texts to write down questions or key concepts to remember [27]. This extra space not only promoted active learning, but also gave readers an area to summarize and synthesize important facts in their own words for future reference and study.

Individual Learning Styles

In addition to attempts to improve organization and word choice in printed materials, a vital but frequently overlooked area of importance is individual learning style. Grebner performed a study examining the effectiveness of an educational intervention tailored to an individual's learning style in comparison to standard health literacy interventions. Health intervention tailored to learning style was indeed shown to increase comprehension compared to standard intervention as measured through statistical comparison of pretesting and post testing of subjects in the learning style tailored intervention group and the standard intervention group. The author suggested a need to apply traditional educational models, such as learning style, to health education in order to improve patient comprehension [28]. While individual learning style may be important, the question then becomes how to identify the learning style of a particular patient. A classic tool to assess learning style is the visual, aural (auditory), read/write, and kinesthetic (VARK) inventory produced by Neil D. Flemming. The assessment consists of a 13 question multiple-choice questionnaire that can be taken and scored quickly to determine learning style [29].

Once an individual's learning style is determined, it is important that appropriate material is provided to them. Visual learners strongly prefer the use of posters, graphs, pictures and diagrams. Moreover, the information should not only have a plethora of pictures but also be well organized and spaced [29]. Auditory learners prefer information presented verbally; thus, clinicians must be sure to discuss any information within printed health materials verbally [29]. Read/Write learners prefer written words and thus printed materials are ideal for them especially when they are presented in list or bullet format in an organized manner as discussed in previous sections of this chapter [29]. Finally, kinesthetic learners learn within the context of what they have previously experienced. Therefore, interactive problems solving, photographs, case studies and real-life examples need to be incorporated into printed materials specific to this learning style [29]. While additional studies are needed to further understand how best to personalize health education materials to individual learning style, we believe this is a promising area of research.

INTERVENTIONS

Clinical Interventions: Tailoring Printed Materials to Individuals

Tailoring printed materials stands in stark contrast to the mass use of a generalized "one size fits all" printed document. Tailoring instead consists of creating an individualized intervention that, ideally, will more effectively impact patient health literacy and health outcomes. Advocates of tailoring suggest that while general health materials may produce modest changes at low cost, they cannot address the myriad of circumstances unique to an individual [30]. The use of tailored printed materials as an intervention has been an avid area of research. Here we focus on tailored interventions used in nutrition and mammography to illustrate the broader applicability of tailored printed materials.

Nutrition

A study performed by the Partners in Prevention-Nutrition program provided individually tailored printed materials to participants with the goals of positively influencing the nutrition practices of adult patients from four North Carolina family practices. The dietary intervention was tailored by assessing the patient's individual stage of nutrition as well as other psychosocial factors. Based on this analysis, a tailored message was mailed to the patient. Compared to the control group, patients receiving tailored messages saw significant decreases in total fat and saturated fat scores. Moreover, a significantly greater number of individuals receiving tailored messages remembered reading the intervention compared to the control group that received a standardized message. The authors suggest that the results show tailored nutrition messages are effective in reducing fat intake and can impact disease prevention [31].

Breast Cancer Prevention

Another study performed by Skinner and colleagues addressed the issue of breast cancer prevention. The intervention consisted of mailing printed materials follow up to patients at two North Carolina family practices and encouraging them to undergo physician-recommended mammography if medically necessary. The messages were tailored based on individual needs and circumstances determined from baseline interviews. The results showed that compared to control groups, women with income below $26,000 and African-American women receiving a tailored intervention follow up by mail were more likely to receive a mammogram if deemed medically necessary compared to the control group. Moreover, tailored letter recipients were significantly more likely to recall receiving and reading the printed materials compared to control [32].

Are Tailored Health Education Materials Effective?

While many studies have suggested the effectiveness of tailored education materials, Kreuter et al. challenges this established view. He contends that a large proportion of recipients do not even recall receiving tailored materials, despite their personalized nature [30, 31, 32]. These observations led to his own investigation into tailored health communication. His study compared overweight adults receiving either a tailored or non-tailored intervention. His analysis was unique in that he determined whether non-tailored material sent to participants was, by chance alone, a good, moderate or poor fit based on behavioral characteristics of the participant. His findings showed that good fitting non-tailored material is as effective as tailored materials for several outcomes. Yet, non-tailored materials that were moderate and poor fitting were not as effective as tailored heath materials. Thus, Kreuter cautions that while tailored materials are effective in many situations they are not more effective in all situations. He suggests that in order to improve tailored materials effectiveness, there is a need for a greater focus on the way tailored materials are developed [33].

Clinical Interventions: Assessing Patient Comprehension of Written Materials

An analysis of patient health literature would be incomplete without assessment of patient comprehension. This can be challenging as patients may not always recognize their lack of understanding and therefore may not voice any concerns regarding their lack of comprehension. As such, the result is inadequate communication between health care provider and patient leading to overall treatment failure. Patient information must be delivered in accordance with individual health literacy, which is often challenging to determine and some patients may attempt to conceal reading impairment or low health literacy due to embarrassment. Furthermore, level of education is a poor indicator of health literacy as a large portion of the public reads several grades lower than the highest achieved level of schooling. A quick screening test to identify those who need special methods of communication is expected to improve patient comprehension.

Assessing Baseline Health Literacy

One of the few tests of patient health literacy is the Short Test of Functional Health Literacy in Adults (STOHFLA). This survey consists of 16 health literacy screening questions which involve asking patients to indicate their level of difficulty in navigating the health care system, completing medical forms, following medication instructions, interacting with providers, and reading appointment slips 33]. The response options are scaled from 0-4. The questions are phrased with non-confrontational wording such as "how often" patients have a problem or "how confident" they feel with aspects of healthcare to encourage more open responses. To test this screening tool, the results of 322 veteran patients were compared with interview findings. The STOHFLA was found to have a high sensitivity for detecting inadequate health literacy but did a poor job of identifying those with marginal health literacy [33]. While this tool needs to be validated on a larger scale in other populations, it serves as a practical assessment of health literacy.

Evaluating Patient Comprehension of Written Materials

The next step is to assess patient comprehension in particular settings. One such example is evaluating patient comprehension of discharge instructions from emergency departments. Emergency departments can be high acuity environments where patients run the risk of being provided incomplete information about their diagnoses and treatments. Lin et al. performed an observational study of 75 adult patients who were discharged with instructions regarding "abdominal pain" and "nausea and vomiting" from a tertiary academic medical center [34]. Patients with altered mental status, developmental delay, and dementia were excluded. The remaining patients were given surveys with open-ended questions regarding their clinical diagnoses, emergency department care, post-discharge instructions, and reasons to return to the hospital. They were also asked to rate their comprehension of these topics on a scale of 1-5 [34]. The patient-reported mean was 4.6. Following the surveys, physicians assessed patient comprehension by scoring patients' responses to questions regarding their illnesses on a scale of 1-5. Next, health care professionals directly evaluated the patients' comprehension of discharge instructions. The physician reported mean assessing patient comprehension was reported to be 3.66 [34]. The patients' self-reported understanding was analyzed against patient evaluation of their understanding and revealed no significant correlation. The results showed that patients' perceptions regarding their comprehension was not in accordance with their actual understanding as assessed by physicians. Patients were found to be least knowledgeable about their diagnoses. The scores of these patients on their STOHFLA also did not correlate with the physician-evaluated level of understanding [34]. This could be a reflection of discharge instructions providing inadequate information resulting in poor comprehension independent of patient health literacy. Further investigation revealed that lapses in patient comprehension were mostly due to omitted information in the discharge instructions.

The teach-back technique can also be employed during the physician-patient interaction to assess patient comprehension while facilitating information transfer. Schillinger et al. conducted a cross-sectional study using audiotape observations of outpatient clinical encounters of 74 adult diabetic patients from 2 primary care sites. The audiotapes were assessed for how frequently new concepts were presented and comprehension was tested by the physician employing teach-back methods [35]. In instances where physicians asked patients to restate medical concepts, incorrect responses were recorded 47% of the time. However, patients of physicians who were subjected to teach-back as part of their visit were found to have lower hemoglobin A_{IC} values reflective of better adherence to physician recommendations [35]. In this setting, direct physician evaluation of patient understanding during clinic visits helped assess patient comprehension and simultaneously promoted improved healthcare practices.

While there are few studies that have assessed patient comprehension, the ones that exist indicate that there is significant room for improvement. Moulton et al. evaluated 60 patients on their comprehension of informed consent forms. The assessment consisted of interviews, a comprehension quiz, and open-ended questions regarding overall clarity of information presented and suggestions for improvement [36]. The comprehension quiz consisted of procedure details, treatment options/risks, and hospital legal implications. The patients were allowed to use the consent form when answering the questions. 46-64% of participants made one or more mistakes [36]. In addition, 58% found the forms to contain confusing words and recommended formatting changes to better highlight key information [36]. About 43% of participants indicated that they had additional questions from the physician, and 82% of participants voiced the desire for additional sources of information [36]. This study is testament to the need for more comprehensible materials for patients.

CONCLUSION

Ultimately, notwithstanding their widespread use, the application of printed health materials for improving health education is in need of great change. Despite the fact that 36% of people in the United States have only basic or below basic healthy literacy skills as determined by the National Assessment of Adult Literacy, the vast majority of printed materials are constructed for individuals at a much higher level of literacy. To improve patient education, the authors of this commentary strongly urge health providers to use the tools suggested including the Flesch-Kincaid Reading Ease test, SMOG Formula, and SAM Trial to tailor printed health materials to a seventh-grade reading level or below. While it is perhaps simpler to develop a "one size fits all" health intervention document, we advise that to best impact the health of patients, it is necessary to invest in the creation of tailored health interventions.

REFERENCES

[1] Hill J. A practical guide to patient education and information giving. *Baillieres Clin Rheumatol.* 1997;11(1):109-127. http://ovidsp.ovid.com/ovidweb.cgi?T=JS&PAGE=reference&D=emed4&NEWS=N&AN=1997094793.

[2] Kessels R. Patients' memory for medical information. *J R Soc Med.* 2003;96(10):520. doi:10.1258/jrsm.96.5.219.

[3] Currie C, Roberts C, Morgan A, Smith R, Settertobulte W, Samdal O. Young people ' s health in context. 2002;(4).

[4] Paul CL, Redman S, Sanson-Fisher RW. Print material content and design: is it relevant to effectiveness? *Health Educ Res.* 2003;18(2):181-190. doi:10.1093/her/18.2.181.

[5] Kirsch IS, Jungeblut A, Jenkins L, Kolstad A. Adult Literacy in America: A First Look at the Results of the National Adult Literacy Survey. *Natl Cent Educ Stat.* 2002:178. doi:NCES 1993-275.

[6] Kutner M, Greenberg E, Jin Y, Paulsen C. Sheida White. 2006.

[7] Nielsen-Bohlman L, Panzer AM, Hamlin B, Kindig DA. Executive Summary. *Heal Lit A Prescr to End Confusion*. 2004:1-25. doi:citeulike-article-id:2393206.

[8] Kincaid JP, Fishburne Jr RP, Rogers RL, Chissom BS. *Derivation of New Readability Formulas (Automated Readability Index, Fog Count and Flesch Reading Ease Formula) for Navy Enlisted Personnel*. DTIC Document; 1975.

[9] Test your document's readability - Office Support. https://support.office.com/en-us/article/Test-your-document-s-readability-0adc0e9a-b3fb-4bde-85f4-c9e88926c6aa. Accessed February 26, 2016.

[10] Hedman AS. Using the SMOG formula to revise a health-related document. *Am J Heal Educ*. 2008;39(1):61-64. doi:10.1080/19325037.2008.10599016.

[11] Shieh C, Hosei B. Printed health information materials: evaluation of readability and suitability. *J Community Health Nurs*. 2008;25(2):73-90. doi:10.1080/07370010802017083.

[12] Suitability assessment of material score sheet | Public Health. https://www.dhhs.tas.gov.au/publichealth/about_us/health_literacy/health_literacy_toolkit/suitability_assessment_of_material_score_sheet. Accessed February 26, 2016.

[13] Hedman AS. Using the SMOG formula to revise a health-related document. *Am J Heal Educ*. 2008;39(1):61-64. doi:10.1080/19325037.2008.10599016.

[14] Klare GR, Buck B. Limitations of the readability formulas. 1954:136-151.

[15] Buxton T. Effective Ways to Improve Health Education Materials. *J Heal Educ*. 1999;30(1):47-61. doi:10.1080/10556699.1999.10628749.

[16] Hoffmann T, Worrall L. Designing effective written health education materials: Considerations for health professionals. *Disabil Rehabil*. 2004;26(19):1166-1173. doi:10.1080/09638280410001724816.

[17] Manning D. Writing readable health messages. *Public Health Rep*. 1981;96(5):464-465. http://www.pubmedcentral.nih.gov/articlerender.fcgi?artid=1424247&tool=pmcentrez&rendertype=abstract.

[18] Meade CD, Smith CF. Readability formulas: Cautions and criteria. *Patient Educ Couns*. 1991;17(2):153-158. doi:10.1016/0738-3991(91)90017-Y.

[19] Dickinson D, Raynor D., Duman M. Patient information leaflets for medicines: using consumer testing to determine the most effective design. *Patient Educ Couns*. 2001;43(2):147-159. doi:10.1016/S0738-3991(00)00156-7.

[20] Wright P. Writing and information design of healthcare materials. *Writ Texts, Process Pract*. 1999:85-98.

[21] Raynor DK. The influence of written information on patient knowledge and adherence to treatment. *Adherence to Treat Med Cond*. 1998:83-111.

[22] Cornett S, Neal W, Ordelt K. In Plain Words: Creating Easy-to-Read Handouts. Children's Healthcare of Atlanta. http://medicine.osu.edu/orgs/ahec/Documents/Toolkit edit.pdf. Accessed July 20, 2016.

[23] Doak CC, Doak LG, Root JH. Teaching patients with low literacy skills. *AJN Am J Nurs*. 1996;96(12):16M.

[24] Mayer G. Enhancing Written Communications to Address Health Literacy. http://www.nursingworld.org/MainMenuCategories/ANAMarketplace/ANAPeriodicals/OJIN/TableofContents/Vol142009/No3Sept09/Enhancing-Written-Communications.html?css=print. Accessed January 24, 2016.

[25] Sanner BM. Are your written materials missing the mark. *J Act Aging*. 2003;2(4):18-24.

[26] Doak LG, Doak CC, Meade CD. Strategies to improve cancer education materials. In: *Oncology Nursing Forum*. Vol 23.; 1996:1305-1312.

[27] Coulter a, Entwistle V, Gilbert D. Sharing decisions with patients: is the information good enough? *Bmj*. 1999;318(7179):318-322. doi:10.1136/bmj.318.7179.318.

[28] Grebner LA. Addressing Learning Style Needs to Improve Effectiveness of Adult Health Literacy Education. *Int J Heal Sci*. 2015;3(1):93-106. doi:10.15640/ijhs.v3n1a6.

[29] Hamilton S. How Do We Assess the Learning Style of Our Patients? *Rehabil Nurs*. 2005;30(4):129-131. http://doi.wiley.com/10.1002/j.2048-7940.2005.tb00095.x. Accessed February 22, 2016.

[30] Kreuter MW, Strecher VJ, Glassman B. One size does not fit all: the case for tailoring print materials. *Annals of behavioral medicine : a publication of the Society of Behavioral Medicine*. doi:10.1007/BF02895958.

[31] Campbell MK, DeVellis BM, Strecher VJ, Ammerman AS, DeVellis RF, Sandler RS. Improving dietary behavior: the effectiveness of tailored messages in primary care settings. *Am J Public Health*.

1994;84(5):783-787. http://www.pubmedcentral.nih.gov/articlerender.fcgi?artid=1615043&tool=pmcentrez&rendertype=abstract. Accessed February 26, 2016.

[32] Skinner CS, Strecher VJ, Hospers H. Physicians' recommendations for mammography: do tailored messages make a difference? *Am J Public Health.* 1994;84(1):43-49. http://www.pubmedcentral.nih.gov/articlerender.fcgi?artid=1614921&tool=pmcentrez&rendertype=abstract. Accessed February 26, 2016.

[33] Kreuter MW, Oswald DL, Bull FC, Clark EM. Are tailored health education materials always more effective than non-tailored materials? *Heal Educ Res.* 2000;15(3):305-315. doi:10.1093/her/15.3.305.

[34] Chew LD, Bradley KA, Boyko EJ. Brief questions to identify patients with inadequate health literacy. *Family medicine.* 2004;36(8):588-594.

[35] Lin MJ, Tirosh AG, Landry A. Examining patient comprehension of emergency department discharge instructions: Who says they understand when they do not? *Internal and emergency medicine.* 2015;10(8):993-1002.

[36] Schillinger D, Piette J, Grumbach K, et al. Closing the loop: physician communication with diabetic patients who have low health literacy. *Archives of internal medicine.* 2003;163(1):83-90.

[37] Manta CJ, Ortiz J, Moulton BW, Sonnad SS. From the Patient Perspective, Consent Forms Fall Short of Providing Information to Guide Decision Making. *Journal of patient safety.* 2016.

APPENDIX

Table. Examples of complex medical jargon and simpler word choice alternatives

More Confusing Medical Word	Simpler Word/Phrase
Immunization	Shots
Edema	Too much fluid
Acute	Sudden
Idiopathic	Unknown cause
Unremarkable	Normal
Hyperlipidemia	High cholesterol
Hypertension	High blood pressure

In: The Evolution of Health Literacy
Editors: N. Agarwal et al.
ISBN: 978-1-53610-602-2

Chapter 3

HEALTH LITERACY: HOW THE INTERNET HAS CHANGED THE WAY PEOPLE RECEIVE HEALTH INFORMATION

Srihari Balasubramanian[1], Jonathan A. Cohen[1], and Jin K. Jung[2], MD
[1]University of Pittsburgh, Pittsburgh, PA, US
[2]Warren Alpert -
Brown University School of Medicine, Providence, RI, US

ABSTRACT

The Internet has quickly become a primary source of information for patients and health conscious individuals alike. Individuals can access enormous amounts of information in a short period. However, the Internet is unique in its ability to utilize visual and auditory elements to enhance the users' learning experience. Despite improvements from traditional health resources such as pamphlets and brochures, the Internet is not devoid of inadequacies. Factors such as language disparities, socioeconomic gaps, and inaccurate information create problems for individuals seeking health information on the web. Throughout this chapter, we broadly explore how the Internet has changed access to health information and its ability to deliver immense content in an engaging and effective manner. However, there are drawbacks of the Internet, both intrinsic and extrinsic, that one must consider when using it as a source of health information.

INTRODUCTION

Since the advent of the Internet, health information has become more widespread and accessible for the regular healthcare consumer. While it was previously relegated solely to textbooks, medical literature, and pamphlets, health information has now greatly increased in its accessibility and availability through the Internet for most Americans. According to Pew Research, 84% of Americans adults use the Internet [1]. This indicates that the vast majority of American adults who are making health decisions for themselves and their family members have an abundance of health information at their fingertips. While this can empower the healthcare decision maker, the abundance of information also has its consequences.

Growth in the amount of accurate health information available to Internet users has been paralleled by a similar rise in the extent of fraudulent and misleading sources of information. The emergence of the Internet as a primary information source has its many benefits as well as challenges. The purpose of this chapter is to explore how the Internet has profoundly affected the means by which healthcare decision makers access and interpret health information, and ultimately, internalize this knowledge to inform their healthcare literacy.

Insufficiency of Traditional Health Resources

Before the Internet emerged as a vital source of healthcare information, people relied most heavily on written information, such as pamphlets, brochures, books, and direct information from healthcare professionals or friends and family. While these sources of information continue to be useful, their availability may be restricted by a myriad of barriers. Many demographics do not have easy access to medical literature or to physicians due to socioeconomic barriers. Furthermore, the target audience of medical books, papers, and articles are assumed to have a certain level of education that enables them to adequately comprehend the information provided. Unfortunately this assumption may lead to inadequate education for certain populations that are disadvantages socioeconomically.

The Internet increases accessibility to health resources through a growing pool of medical information. It permits instantaneous health answers and empowers patients by ensuring appropriate healthcare autonomy. Information is presented on the Internet in a variety of fashions that cater to difference demographics regardless of cultural, economic, or social differences.

Internet as a Resource for Health Information

The Internet is an enormous resource for acquiring health information, and many people in the United States use it for precisely that. A study conducted by Hesse et al. in 2005 uncovered that 64% of the people who used the Internet searched for health information [2]. The majority of Internet users included patients who wanted to know what their symptoms meant and physicians who wanted to stay informed on the new breakthroughs in their fields. [3]. A major reason that the Internet is able to bridge several gaps in health literacy is due to its availability and its size. With well over 70,000 websites dedicated to health information, the Internet has an incredible amount of medical knowledge stored on it – from scholarly articles to websites with different forms of multimedia including videos, PowerPoints, and interactive presentations [4, 5]. To best utilize these online resources and optimize the user experience, websites are intentionally designed to be user-friendly, interactive, and easy to manipulate. This interface helps people navigate through the various resources and extract relevant health information with ease.

Visual Cues

A major point of distinction between traditional health information resources and the Internet is the mechanisms of interaction with the information. While sifting through traditional methods of health literacy, communication relies heavily on written cues. However, navigating through the Internet can be augmented with the use of visual cues. A webpage has the capability of offering a complete visual experience. This is enabled by the use of different multimedia such as images, charts, and videos that serve as valuable education modalities for patients

The use of images serves as an effective means for transmitting health information to patients. Health communication materials that contain pictures receive considerably more attention than those without pictures [6]. Additionally, a study demonstrated that patients were significantly more likely to read and remember handouts with pictures than those without. These study subjects had improved retention of health information when they were presented with pictures [6]. This notion can be applied to verbal methods of communication as well. When a group of people were given health information with accompanying visual aids, they responded with more accurate and abundant recall than the group that were given health instructions alone. This has powerful implications as it demonstrates that patients more effectively comprehend health information that is accompanied by visual cues [7].

When this concept is extended to the Internet, one can appreciate why health communication through this channel is such a powerful tool. Webpages are designed to be interactive, consisting of pictures, diagrams, voiceovers, videos and animations intended to engage users and enhance the learning experience. Despite the diverse options and flexibility of web design, developing effective online health resources is not trivial. It is important to design effective webpages that are easy to navigate and clearly explain their purpose.

Designing Effective Webpages

Due to the prevalence of electronic health records throughout the healthcare industry, it is becoming easier for patients to access their records through online portals. These portals are typically available through the websites of their physician, which makes it imperative that the webpages be user friendly and culturally sensitive [8].

The most useful type of webpage will contain the following characteristics:

- Simple Language
- Pictures with Captions
- Videos
- Table of Contents
- Links to Additional Information

Regardless of the content of the webpage, it is important that the website be simple. There should not be superfluous information or too much detail on the webpage – only the most pertinent and important information should be present. Patients generally find a webpage more satisfying if the language is simple and it contains more pictures [9]. Coupled with evidence that consumers best recall health information with pictures and text, this suggests that a simple picture with a concise caption is an ideal visual aid in a webpage [9, 10].

New Challenges Posed by the Internet on Health Literacy

Despite several noted advantages of delivering health content via the Internet, a new set of challenges arises with this technology. First, patients who obtain health information online may receive too much exposure and develop incorrect perceptions of knowledge pertaining to a specific health subject. Although the patients experience symptoms of medical ailments, many patients may lack adequate expertise to diagnose themselves. This may prove problematic as they turn to online health information to 'self-diagnose' themselves—whether accurate or not—through the click of a button. The Internet may be filled with useful, evidence-based information; however, physicians require extensive education to be licensed, and, thus, should bear the responsibility of interpreting symptoms and diagnosing patients.

Access

While the Internet does increase the availability of health information, it does not completely erase the issue of access. Nationwide, 11.9% of households with median incomes of less than $34,783 survive without broadband access. This number becomes even more significant when compared with the 2.6% of households with incomes of $80,694 or greater that do not have access to broadband. [11]. Low income and rural communities without a high-speed connection or computers continue to be at a major disadvantage. They face similar accessibility problems as they faced with traditional healthcare resources, which can cause them to turn a blind eye to their health.

Technological Literacy

Though these accessibility issues can be partially allayed with widespread public availability of computers, another challenge arises: technological literacy. In order to properly navigate the Internet, users must have a certain level of computer experience and technological literacy. This requirement further narrows the groups of people who can comfortably access vital health information on the Internet, often excluding citizens that are older and at a lower socioeconomic level [12]. As people become increasingly reliant on the Internet for health information, those who are burdened by socioeconomic and age-related barriers to access may be discouraged from accessing health information. Furthermore, patients from low-income areas may lack technological literacy, and technology may thus be underutilized [13].

Language

For populations that are not affected by the aforementioned socioeconomic barriers, there still remains another critical challenge: language. As the world is becoming increasingly globalized, there are millions of people who are living in a country in which the language spoken is not their native tongue. This is particularly true in the United States. Naturally, this creates difficulty for doctors when they communicate health information to their patients. Consequently, this language barrier may drive immigrant communities to seek additional health information from the Internet. However, once they get on the Internet, they potentially face the same language difficulties that they experience with their English-speaking physicians. In a 2014 survey, English represented over 50% of the top 10 million webpages visited. English is also the most common language that is used by Internet users [14]. This means that the easiest and most available websites are those written in English. For immigrant communities and communities without access to quality education, this can be a major issue. Limited English proficiency negatively impacts patient safety, so any miscomprehension of health information such as medication dosing and dietary restrictions put patients at risk [15]. An illustration of this is an English as Second Language (ESL) patient that attempts to read a prescription written in English. If this patient tries to access instructional information on the Internet, there is a greater chance that she will find the information she is looking for on a webpage written in English as opposed to her native tongue. In this case, even if she finds the information, she will likely have a hard time piecing the information together in English, and therefore still faces the imminent possibility of giving herself an incorrect dosage. This hypothetical example illustrates how many communities who speak and write English as a second language who do have access to the Internet and do not face the economic barriers to computer usage may still be inhibited from finding useful health information.

Quality Control

Although the Internet can empower patients, it oftentimes contains incorrect information misinforming patients of their actual healthcare needs. Furthermore, there is no standard quality check, which makes it difficult for patients to evaluate the accuracy of the information they come across [16]. Although this challenge does exist with traditional sources of health information, it is amplified with the ubiquity of the Internet. The Internet is open for anyone and everyone to create – this has merits and consequences. Because there is relatively little regulation on what types of health information can be written on the Internet, any person—even a biased patient who had a negative healthcare experience—can create a website containing false or anecdotal health information for all to access [5]. If a patient consults the Internet and comes across sensible advice, she may call into question the decision-making and diagnosis of the doctor without warrant [17]. This may place the patient's well being at risk and is a direct consequence of unregulated, false health information.

In addition to webpages with blatantly false information, webpages with accurate, factual information have the ability to lead consumers of healthcare astray. As described elsewhere, many health websites are written at a much higher reading level than the 3rd to 7th grade level as recommended by the American Medical Association and the National Institutes of Health. This increases the difficulty of reading and comprehending different illnesses, diagnoses, and prescriptions, and overwhelms patients with medical jargon. Online health resources are not personalized. That is, they are often inundated with highly technical, non-essential information that exceeds the needs of the patients. Due to the accumulation of information, extracting pertinent and valid details is becoming increasingly difficult. It makes health information difficult to sift through and put meaning behind [18]. As a result, patients retain little information and develop an incomplete fund of medical knowledge. This acts as another barrier for patients.

CONCLUSION

The Internet is a powerful tool to improve health literacy and help patients take an active role in their health. However, the Internet poses many challenges such as unverified, non-peer-reviewed information and can be difficult for patients from lower socioeconomic groups and with language difficulties to access and understand. The Internet will undoubtedly continue to grow as a major source of healthcare information, and its ability to deliver engaging content can be used as a tool to strengthen the physician-patient relationship.

REFERENCES

[1] Perrin, A, Duggan M. Americans' Internet Access: 2000-2015. 2015; http://www.pewInternet.org/2015/06/26/americans-Internet-access-2000-2015/. Accessed September 13, 2016.

[2] Hesse BW, Nelson DE, Kreps GL, et al. Trust and sources of health information: The impact of the Internet and its implications for health care providers: findings from the first health information national trends survey. *Archives of Internal Medicine.* 2005;165(22):2618-2624.

[3] Tang H, Ng JHK. Googling for a diagnosis—use of Google as a diagnostic aid: Internet based study. *BMJ.* 2006;333(7579):1143.

[4] Grandinetti DA. Doctors and the Web. Help your patients surf the Net safely. *Medical Economics.3//2000; 77(5): 186-8, 194-6, 201.*

[5] Richards B, Colman AW, Hollingsworth RA. The current and future role of the Internet in patient education. *Int J Med Inform.* 06// 1998;50(1-3):279-285.

[6] Houts PS, Doak CC, Doak LG, Loscalzo MJ. The role of pictures in improving health communication: A review of research on attention, comprehension, recall, and adherence. *Patient Education and Counseling.* 5// 2006;61(2):173-190.

[7] Houts PS, Witmer JT, Egeth HE, Loscalzo MJ, Zabora JR. Using pictographs to enhance recall of spoken medical instructions II. *Patient Education and Counseling.* 6// 2001;43(3):231-242.

[8] Egbert N, Nanna, K. Health Literacy: Challenges and Strategies. *OJIN: The Online Journal of Issues in Nursing.* 2009;14(3).

[9] van Weert JCM, van Noort G, Bol N, van Dijk L, Tates K, Jansen J. Tailored information for cancer patients on the Internet: Effects of visual cues and language complexity on information recall and satisfaction. *Patient Education and Counseling.*84(3):368-378.

[10] Schmidt-Weigand F KA, Glowalla U. A closer look at split visual attention in system- and self-paced instruction in multimedia learning. . *Learning and Instruction.* 2010;20(2):100-110.

[11] Holmes A, Bell Fox E, Wieder B, Zubak-Skees C. Rich people have access to high-speed Internet; many poor people still don't; May 12, 2016; https://www.publicintegrity.org/2016/05/12/19659/rich-people-have-access-high-speed-internet-many-poor-people-still-dont/ . Accessed December 12, 2016.

[12] Ybarra M, Suman M. Reasons, assessments and actions taken: sex and age differences in uses of Internet health information. *Health Education Research.* June 1, 2008 2008;23(3):512-521.

[13] Jensen JD, King, A. J., Davis, L. A., Guntzviller, L. M. Utilization of Internet technology by low-income adults: The role of health literacy, health numeracy, and computer assistance. *Journal of Aging and Health.* 2010;22(6):804-826.

[14] Usage of content languages for websites. 2016; https://w3techs.com/technologies/overview/content_language/all. Accessed September 13, 2016.

[15] Derose PK, Escarce JJ, Lurie N. Immigrants And Healthcare: Sources of Vulnerability. *Health Affairs*. 2007. 26(5): 1258-68.

[16] Hernandez, Lyla M. *Health Literacy: Improving Health, Health Systems, and Health Policy around the World: Workshop Summary*. N.p.: n.p., n.d. Print.

[17] Rice RE. Influences, usage, and outcomes of Internet health information searching: Multivariate results from the Pew surveys. *International Journal of Medical Informatics*. 2006. 75(1): 8-28.

[18] C. S. Health literacy: concept analysis. *J Adv Nurs Journal of Advanced Nursing.* 2005;50(6):633-640.

In: The Evolution of Health Literacy
Editors: N. Agarwal et al.
ISBN: 978-1-53610-602-2

Chapter 4

METRICS FOR ASSESSMENT OF ONLINE PATIENT EDUCATION MATERIALS

Rafey A. Feroze[1] and Michael M. McDowell, MD[2]
[1]University of Pittsburgh School of Medicine, Pittsburgh, PA US
[2]Department of Neurological Surgery, University of Pittsburgh Medical Center, Pittsburgh, PA, US

ABSTRACT

With the advent of the digital age, the amount of patient health information available online has increased dramatically. However, such information is of low utility unless it is designed to suit the level and needs of the general public. Online health information has been evaluated using various metrics that assess readability, accessiblity, usability, and reliability. These criteria together provide an understanding of the degree to which a typical user can interact with the material presented. Across numerous sources, the readability of patient health literature was found to be higher than the reading level of the general American populace. Standards for improving health website accessiblity exist and have been applied with room for improvement. Usability is determined by evaluation of simulated users regarding the ease of obtaining lasting knowledge from a source. A wide range of variability exists in usability and reliability of online patient health information. Consideration of all four of these aspects is necessary in improving quality of patient health literature.

INTRODUCTION

The increasing sophistication and specialization in medicine in the past few decades has made health literacy a crucial part of patient care. Health literacy has been defined as “the degree to which individuals have the capacity to obtain, process, and understand basic health information and services needed to make appropriate health decisions”[1]. With the advent of more complex medications and treatments protocols, patient knowledge regarding their diseases and therapies is necessary to establish compliance and efficacy. In addition, studies have shown a positive effect on the physician-patient relationship when patients actively participate in their treatment [2].

Technology advancement has allowed for digitalized storage and distribution of large amounts of health information. Studies show that 63% of U.S. Internet users and 71% of European Internet users rely on online health resources for information [3, 4]. While the increased access to health information has created a tremendous potential benefit in allowing patients and their families to better understand medical problems and treatments, such information must be accurate, up to date, and presented in a manner comprehensible to those without medical training.

The complexity of health information and the large number of resources available are often overwhelming to a lay audience. As a result, patients with low health literacy suffer from reduced knowledge about their conditions. The American Medical Association (AMA) has cited health literacy as the strongest independent predictor of health status and correlated a lower level of health literacy to a greater risk of hospitalization [5]. Patients with low health literacy have also been shown to have reduced treatment compliance and higher mortality [6]. From an economic standpoint, patients with low health literacy incur four times more in medical expenses compared to their more health literate counterparts [7]. On a national scale, the U.S. Department of Health and Human Services Office of Disease Prevention and Health Promotion has estimated that poor health literacy costs the U.S. economy 106-236 billion dollars annually [8]. Access to easily understood health information to at risk patients is a crucial part of combating this problem.

Evaluation of healthcare information involves ensuring its readability, reliability, usability, and accessibility with respect to patients. With increased awareness regarding the importance of health literacy, numerous studies have been conducted to assess these categories in health information sources. This chapter outlines the various methods and metrics employed to evaluate patient health literature and how they can be used to improve dissemination of health information.

READABILITY

Readability is a key aspect of literacy and largely refers to the ease with which written materials can be comprehended. The readability of health education materials should be commensurate to the health literacy of the general populace and alternate versions of variable difficulty are recommended. Reading material is considered easy to read when below a sixth grade level, of average difficulty when between the seventh and ninth grade reading level, and difficult when above the ninth grade reading level [9]. The average reading level of American adults has been reported to be between the seventh and eighth grade levels. Furthermore, the average American adult reads 3-5 grades below their highest grade of schooling [9]. Therefore, the AMA and National Institutes of Health (NIH) recommend designing patient education materials to be between the third and seventh grade reading levels [5]. Despite these literacy limitations, websites of many national organizations that provide health information for answering patient questions present material at a level of comprehension that is higher than the recommended guidelines [10, 11, 12].

Previous studies have focused on assessing the readability of patient education materials. Various readability scales have been used to analyze health information text. These scales involve analysis of the number of letters/syllables in words and sentence structure in a body of text. Commonly used readability scales include the Coleman-Liau Index, Flesch-Kincaid Grade Level, Flesch Reading Ease scale, FORCAST Formula, Fry Graph, Gunning Fog Index, New Dale-Chall scale, New Fog Count, Raygor Readability Estimate, and the SMOG Readability Formula [13]. Nine of these scales provide a readability grade that correlates with the academic grade level that is most likely needed to understand the material. The Flesch Reading Ease scale provides a result from 0-100 with a score of 0-30 indicating very difficult; 30-50, difficult; 50-60, fairly difficult; 60-70, standard; 70-80, fairly easy; 80-90, easy; and 90-100, very easy [13]. The scores from the nine readability metrics that provide a grade level can be averaged together to provide a mean score for a certain text.

Studies utilizing these scales have shown that an overwhelming majority of articles are too difficult for the average American and of a higher readability than the recommended guidelines. For example, a study evaluating 339 patient education materials from ophthalmologic association websites showed readability scores ranging from 8.2 to 18.7 grade levels using the indexes including the Flesch Kincaid Grade Level, Gunning Fog Index, and Raygor Readabilty Estimate, to name a few [5]. Similarly, another study evaluating information from the European Society of Radiology website, which evaluated 41 articles and averaged the results across the nine readability scales, reported a mean grade level of 13.0 ±1.6 with a range of 10.8 and 17.2 [8]. In this case, even the article with the lowest readability would be deemed far too difficult to read in regards to the AMA and NIH recommendations. A study using the New Dale-Chall readability test comparing the readability of patient education material from national society websites of 16 medical specialties indicated that only dermatology, family medicine, and obstetrics and gynecology patient education materials were close to the average American adult reading level [12]. These high readability scores across many specialties epitomize the breadth of this problem and the need for more comprehensible patient education materials.

While most health education literature has compared the difficulty of patient education materials to the reading level of the average American, there are far fewer studies that address the even greater concern for certain subsets of patients with reading comprehension skills below the general populace. These groups of patients may be associated with particular health problems. For example, patients who suffer from traumatic brain injury, dementia, autism, or general cognitive impairment are likely to have limited reading comprehension abilities. Many of these patients may undergo neurological rehabilitation and require information presented in a simpler way than healthier individuals without cognitive or neurological deficits. However, a study showed that neurological surgery rehabilitation patient education material, evaluated using the Flesch Reading Ease Scale and the Flesch-Kincaid Grade Level, were of a higher reading level than that of the average American let alone suitable for those with impaired cognitive abilities [14]. Even more specialized health education resources need to be designed corresponding to the reading level of this subgroup of patients.

Another example of a specialized group of patients is those from economically impoverished and medically underserved populations who have lower than average literacy but are disproportionally burdened by lifestyle related diseases such as diabetes and cardiovascular disease.[15] Evaluation of patient education information from the American Heart Association and American Diabetes Association showed some documents with appropriate grade levels ($\leq 5^{th}$ grade), but most documents were above the recommended guidelines. Some sentences were even found to be of grade levels as high as 23-24 [15]. Given that less education and poverty are correlated with low health literacy [16], more readable patient education materials must be designed for informing underserved populations.

While the readability scales mentioned above are a quick and easy way to determine whether a text is too difficult for the general public, they suffer from some major limitations. Since most of them use number of syllables per word, number of words per sentence, and sentence structure to determine readability, the content of the material is not evaluated. Therefore, small words that are still considered medical jargon, such as "edema" or "ileum" would not be added to the calculated complexity. Simultaneously, polysyllabic words such as "consciousness" or "medication" that are part of common parlance would wrongfully increase the readability. The word order also contributes to the readability and is not evaluated by the aforementioned scales. Finally, the readability indexes do not take page layout, images, videos, or forms of multimedia supplementation into consideration when evaluating medical information.

There are guidelines created by the AMA, NIH, and the Centers for Disease Control and Prevention on how to write healthcare patient information in a way that is comprehensible to the general American population. The patient education resources available at the American Academy of Family Physicians website have been shown to be at a level that is in accordance with the NIH and AMA guidelines [12]. However, as indicated above and in numerous other instances in patient health literature, the webpages of most major medical societies contain material that is of a higher reading level than the gerenal populace. Given that healthcare professionals with years of medical training and experience with writing literature for colleagues are writing patient education materials, the high reading levels associated with the articles is not surprising [17]. Nevertheless, a lower reading level is expected to be more easily comprehensible to the general public and thereby more effective in providing valuable patient information and advancing health literacy.

ACCESSIBILITY

Accessibility refers to whether a large portion of the population can obtain and use certain information. Websites are now required by the United States and many other countries to abide by accessibility requirements outlined by the World Wide Web Consortium (W3C) and Bobby standards [18]. These standards comprise a list of guidelines which are in place to help web developers in designing web content accessible to people with disabilities such as not being able to see, hear, move a keyboard/mouse, or difficulty reading and comprehending text. The guidelines also take into account how some users may have a text-only screen, small screen, or slow Internet connection. Design solutions for such concerns are provided as part of the standards.

The W3C guidelines recommend: making texts/graphics understandable without color, using tools that facilitate interpretation of abbreviated or foreign text, developing websites that allow user interface with a variety of input devices, providing clear navigation mechanisms, ensuring that documents are clear and simple, and validating accessibility with automatic tools and human review [19]. Furthermore, the W3C guidelines also encourage providing appropriate alternatives to visual content such as pre-recorded audio, synthesized text, braille displays, text equivalents for multimedia content, and substitutes to compensate for cognitive disabilities, visual disabilities, and deafness in order to make health information more accessible to patients [19]. The presence of non-text equivalents can also help compensate for aforementioned readability issues. Additionally, providing control of time-sensitive content such as blinking and moving objects on a website is beneficial to patients who process information slowly or are prone to seizures from such triggers. Such strategies are likely to make websites more accessible to all users and should be followed for patient education materials.

A validated method of evaluating healthcare websites called the LIDA tool has been used to determine the accessibility, usability and reliability. It contains 41 questions that provide a percentage for each of the three categories. These questions can be answered by a series of evaluators who are blinded to each other's scores and the results are averaged to determine a final score [18]. The accessibility portion tests whether a website adheres to the W3C standards described above and whether the health information is readily available without subscriptions or lengthy sign in procedures. Studies evaluating accessibility of online patient information also test if websites are compatible with various browsers and whether the HTML code is up-to-date [20]. LIDA testing of patient education material from the American Academy of Orthopedic Surgeons and Pediatric Orthopedic Society of North America resulted in accessibility scores of 78% and 66%, respectively [18]. Similarly, a study evaluating 250 websites regarding tonsillectomies, obtained from five different Internet search engines, reported an average accessibility score of

66.7% using LIDA testing [20]. All of these scores are considered to be within the moderate range, indicating considerable success in providing accessible patient information with room for further improvement.

USABILITY

Unlike readability which evaluates the level of sophistication of presented text, usability encompasses a holistic view of the ease at which user can interact with and absorb the information presented. This may include many factors such as the design of a webpage, the ratio of textual information to multimedia supplementation, engage-ability with the user, and ease of navigation. Pertinent factors can range from the color and font used to the organization of the information presented. For example, an interactive series of schematics and diagrams which require the user to pick and choose the relevant information would enhance the usability in comparison to a large amount of text information presented without any clear guidance. Unlike the readability metrics described above, usability testing involves measuring end-user performance in controlled situations. Video analysis of simulated end-users to determine time taken to perform various task and logging of their interactions with the information can help evaluate usability [21]. Simulated users often answer a set of questions pertaining to their experience. Therefore, it is important to have a variety of individuals with different educational backgrounds, who represent the target audience, involved in the usability testing to help prevent selection bias.

The LIDA tool has been used to evaluate the usability of patient health information and gives a percentage score. Evaluation of the American Association of Orthopedic Surgery and Pediatric Orthopedic Society of North American websites reported usability scores of 84% and 73%, respectively [18]. The tonsillectomy study mentioned above reported an average 53.7% usability score, with the majority of webpages falling in the moderate score group [20]. Failure of these websites to engage the users and interact with their audience prevented them from receiving higher scores. As a result, users are unlikely to learn and retain a significant amount of valuable health information.

The addition of visual aids to textual information has been shown to enhance the usability of health information. A study showed 92-94% of low literacy patients found pill cards, which depict medication regimen with images and icons, to be easy to understand and helpful for remembering important medication information [22]. A study aiming to develop a web-based education system for low-literate parents of neonatal patients suffering from patent ductus arteriosus used text at the 5th grade readability level coupled with active voiced conversational language in short sentences, substituted technical words for simpler language where possible, added voice-recorded sound files to text elements that were considered difficult, and supplemented text with pictographs illustrating recommended tasks involving the parent and child [21]. To cater to a low literate audience, the authors limited topics to 3 per screen, kept pages short and concise, used subheading and bullet points, used large buttons that were easy to identify, and limited the use of multiple windows, drop down menus, and scroll bars. As a result, the education system received a mean score of 4.52 on a 0-5 scale of 'Perceived Ease of Use and Usefulness.' The study participants indicated that the readability was appropriate, that the pictographs were helpful in conveying information, and that the voice recordings were the most-liked feature. In addition, the participants felt that photographs would be more relatable than pictographs and that too many pop-ups or hypertext links were distracting [21]. A moderate amount of multimedia supplementation is a proven way to enhance usability of patient information. Large amounts of text without multimedia clarification forces readers to reconstruct mental images without adequate experience [23]. The use of appropriate images to illustrate textual information can make it easier for lower literacy patients and family members to make visual associations and enhance their understanding of medication and treatments, thereby increasing their compliance and lowering hospitalization, disease, and mortality.

Reliability

Reliable information is expected to be accurate, evidence-based, relevant, comprehensive, unbiased, and up-to-date. Given that the information presented to patients guides decisions that directly impact their health, reliability is a crucial factor in patient health literature. Reliability can be ensured by experts who organize the patient health information, regularly update websites to keep up with advances in the medical field, comprehensively review all background information to be inclusive, adequately cite all health information sources used, and declare sponsorship or potential conflicts of interests [20]. However, no standards exist regarding reliability of health information on the Internet, resulting in potentially misleading information sources. Furthermore, there is no service which oversees the quality of patient health literature presented on the Internet and assigns penalties when unreliable information is disseminated.

LIDA analysis of the orthopedic websites described above showed high mean reliability scores of 85-87%, and the information presented was found to be current and unbiased. The information was also supported with links from outside groups, and the identities of authors were easily verified. However, these websites were unable to achieve higher scores due to questionable funding sources and low frequency with which information was updated [18].

While the reliability of these websites was found to be high, some other studies did not report similar scores. The tonsillectomy study mentioned above reported average reliability scores of 33.3% using the LIDA test [20]. A study on health information websites for patients regarding peripheral vascular disease, in which the authors used a customized method of scoring websites based on rating from expert observers, showed that 32% of the evaluated webpages contained misleading or non-conventional treatment information while only 23% presented material pertinent to patient education. These results are surprising given that 67.8% of the authors were found to be of an academic or biomedical background [17].

Such discrepancies may result from a significant amount of information encountered on the Internet being commercially motivated or aiming to advance a new area of research, rather than providing the most feasible medical advice for patients. A study evaluating lumbar disc herniation information on the Internet indicates that 34.3% of evaluated websites sought secondary commercial gain [24]. While the use of the Internet to advance commercial intentions of medical agencies is not in itself a violation and should be permitted, it is important to note that it is easy for the general public to confuse commercially motivated information with conventional medical practice. Therefore, an increased effort towards specifying which information is suitable for patients and including disclaimers regarding the impact of commercial literature on patients' health decisions should be made.

Most of the patient information websites do not include sections for user feedback and comments. Crowdsourcing can be tricky as it is challenging to regulate the type of information that is included. However, opinions from similar users regarding the quality of information and their resulting experiences can help patients formulate more confident conclusions, thereby increasing the usefulness of the website. Such a system has been incorporated in numerous Internet based services and is a possible avenue to incorporate in patient information websites.

A handful of reports indicate low reliability of patient health information; however, publication bias may play a role. Overall, there are few studies available evaluating the reliability of patient information, making it difficult to draw general conclusions [20]. Broad use of a standardized method, such as the LIDA tool, is needed to further assess the reliability of the majority of patient-focused literature.

CONCLUSION

While the Internet has certainly made health literature accessible to the masses, it currently suffers from several limitations in dispersing patient oriented information. Systematic evaluation of existing patient health literature is difficult but the first step toward improving quality of such information. Many such studies have been conducted and highlight the types of improvements needed in readability, accessibility, and usability of patient health literature. It is well-established that most patient-oriented health literature is of too high a reading level and difficult to be comprehensible to the general public; this literature must be redesigned to be more easily understandable, interactive with the user, and accessible to those with disabilities. While standardized guidelines exist for accessibility of websites, there are no such regulations governing reliability and usability of patient health information. Improvements in these areas are expected to improve patient health literacy.

REFERENCES

[1] Institute of Medicine Committee on Health L. In: Nielsen-Bohlman L, Panzer A. M., Kindig D. A., eds. *Health Literacy: A Prescription to End Confusion*. Washington (DC): National Academies Press (US) Copyright 2004 by the National Academy of Sciences. All rights reserved; 2004.

[2] McMullan M. Patients using the Internet to obtain health information: how this affects the patient-health professional relationship. *Patient education and counseling*. 2006; 63(1-2):24-28.

[3] Andreassen H. K., Bujnowska-Fedak MM, Chronaki CE, et al. European citizens' use of E-health services: a study of seven countries. *BMC public health*. 2007; 7:53.

[4] Hesse B. W., Nelson D. E., Kreps G. L., et al. Trust and sources of health information: the impact of the Internet and its implications for healthcare providers: findings from the first Health Information National Trends Survey. *Archives of internal medicine.* 2005; 165 (22):2618-2624.

[5] Huang G., Fang C. H., Agarwal N., Bhagat N., Eloy J. A., Langer P. D. Assessment of online patient education materials from major ophthalmologic associations. *JAMA ophthalmology.* 2015; 133(4):449-454.

[6] Health literacy: report of the Council on Scientific Affairs. Ad Hoc Committee on Health Literacy for the Council on Scientific Affairs, American Medical Association. *Jama.* 1999; 281 (6):552-557.

[7] Weiss B. D., Blanchard J. S., McGee D. L., et al. Illiteracy among Medicaid recipients and its relationship to healthcare costs. *Journal of healthcare for the poor and underserved.* 1994; 5(2):99-111.

[8] Hansberry D. R., Agarwal N., Baker S. R. Health literacy and online educational resources: an opportunity to educate patients. *AJR. American journal of roentgenology.* 2014; 204(1):111-116.

[9] Walsh T. M., Volsko T. A. Readability assessment of Internet-based consumer health information. *Respiratory care.* 2008; 53 (10):1310-1315.

[10] Kasabwala K., Misra P., Hansberry D. R., et al. Readability assessment of the American Rhinologic Society patient education materials. *International forum of allergy and rhinology.* 2012; 3 (4):325-333.

[11] Misra P., Agarwal N., Kasabwala K., Hansberry D. R., Setzen M., Eloy J. A. Readability analysis of healthcare-oriented education resources from the American Academy of Facial Plastic and Reconstructive Surgery. *The Laryngoscope.* 2012; 123 (1):90-96.

[12] Agarwal N., Hansberry D. R., Sabourin V., Tomei K. L., Prestigiacomo C. J. A comparative analysis of the quality of patient education materials from medical specialties. *JAMA Intern Med.* Vol 173. United States2013:1257-1259.

[13] Hansberry DR, John A, John E, Agarwal N, Gonzales SF, Baker SR. A critical review of the readability of online patient education resources from RadiologyInfo.Org. *AJR. American journal of roentgenology.* 2014; 202 (3):566-575.

[14] Agarwal N., Sarris C., Hansberry D. R., Lin M. J., Barrese J. C., Prestigiacomo C. J. Quality of patient education materials for

rehabilitation after neurological surgery. *NeuroRehabilitation.* 2013; 32(4):817-821.

[15] Hill-Briggs F., Smith A. S. Evaluation of diabetes and cardiovascular disease print patient education materials for use with low-health literate populations. *Diabetes care.* 2008; 31 (4):667-671.

[16] Cutilli C. C., Bennett I. M. Understanding the Health Literacy of America Results of the National Assessment of Adult Literacy. *Orthop Nurs.* 2009; 28 (1):27-34.

[17] Soot L. C., Moneta G. L., Edwards J. M. Vascular surgery and the Internet: a poor source of patient-oriented information. *Journal of vascular surgery.* 1999; 30 (1):84-91.

[18] Feghhi DP, Komlos D, Agarwal N, Sabharwal S. Quality of online pediatric orthopaedic education materials. *The Journal of bone and joint surgery. American volume.* 2014;96 (23):e194.

[19] Henry S. W3C web accessiblity initiative. *Introduction to Web Accessiblity.*

[20] Roshan A., Agarwal S., England R. Role of Information Available Over the Internet: What are the Parents of Children Undergoing Tonsillectomy Likely to Find? *Ann R Coll Surg Engl.* 2008; 90 (7):601-605.

[21] Choi J., Bakken S. Web-based education for low-literate parents in Neonatal Intensive Care Unit: development of a website and heuristic evaluation and usability testing. *International journal of medical informatics.* 2010; 79 (8):565-575.

[22] Kripalani S, Robertson R, Love-Ghaffari MH, et al. Development of an illustrated medication schedule as a low-literacy patient education tool. *Patient education and counseling.* 2007; 66 (3):368-377.

[23] Mayer R. Multimedia aids to problem-solving transfer ☆. 1999; 31(7):611–623.

[24] Greene DL, Appel AJ, Reinert SE, Palumbo MA. Lumbar disc herniation: evaluation of information on the Internet. *Spine.* 2005; 30(7):826-829.

In: The Evolution of Health Literacy
Editors: N. Agarwal et al.
ISBN: 978-1-53610-602-2

Chapter 5

METHODS AND IMPACT OF IMPROVING HEALTH LITERACY

Jasmine Kashkoush[1], Ahmed Kashkoush[2] and Kamil W. Nowicki[3], MD, PhD
[1]University of South Florida Morsani College of Medicine, Tampa, FL, US
[2]University of Pittsburgh School of Medicine, Pittsburgh, PA US
[3]Department of Neurological Surgery, University of Pittsburgh Medical Center, Pittsburgh, PA, US

ABSTRACT

Patients heavily rely on physician-provided healthcare information. When inadequate, patients seek outside sources, such as the Internet to increase their knowledge on their medical management. Although these sources have the potential to positively affect patient outcomes, they must be accurate and easily understood by a medically illiterate audience. Health literacy is the ability to understand health-related information to make appropriate informed medical decisions. By increasing health literacy levels through engaged physician-patient interactions, enhanced accuracy and validity of sources, and personalized care, we can empower patients when making informed healthcare decisions and improve patient outcomes.

1. INTRODUCTION

Every day patients make decisions regarding their health. These decisions span from routine choices such as diet to more serious decisions such as those regarding disease management. Most patients are unfamiliar with the numerous medical specialties and this poses a challenge when making choices that impact an individual's health. Patients want to make effective, informed decisions that adhere to their values. The decision-making process may become very complicated in the absence of adequate patient education.

Shared decision making, by combining the knowledge of a physician and the desires of a patient, helps alleviate some of the obstacles caused by patient misinformation. By establishing a mutual agenda between a patient and a physician, shared decision making empowers individuals as they become more involved in their health. However, physicians are not always accessible nor do they always explain concepts in plain language that patients can understand. As patients often get lost in the medical jargon that physicians relay, they frequently seek outside resources, such as the Internet, to gain a better understanding of unfamiliar concepts. Hesse et al., reported that 63% of the U.S. adult population used the Internet and that 64% of these Internet users reported using the Internet for health information for themselves or others [62]. However, there is a growing apprehension that these resources are providing unreliable and even, inaccurate health information, putting an individual's health at risk. The Internet has the potential to eliminate barriers to access information for patients; however, this can only occur if online material can be read and understood by users with various levels of medical sophistication [31].

Individuals with limited health literacy are at a disadvantage when dealing with the healthcare system. Although they are able to attend appointments and understand very basic information provided in pamphlets, these individuals are unable to understand common medical terms that clinicians use on a daily basis such as "colon," "blood in the stool," "screening test," and "lesion." [5]. In one study, one in four women who reported that they knew what a mammogram was, when asked, turned out not to know [6]. The lack of patient health literacy widens the gap of knowledge between a physician and a patient, as patients may not be informing their caregivers when they do not understand certain concepts. Thus, caregivers may be overestimating the literacy and health literacy levels of their patients. Even highly literate, well-educated individuals struggle to understand what their clinician is telling them, as clinicians often use vocabulary and concepts unfamiliar to those without a medical background [4]. In one such report, even an obstetrician related being unable to fully comprehend his orthopedist's explanations [4]. If physicians of different specialties cannot even fully comprehend each other, it makes it very unlikely that patients with no or little medical background will.

Limited health literacy poses a risk to patient outcomes. When investigating predictors of future health status, studies have shown health literacy to be the strongest predictor, even greater than income, employment status, education level, and racial or ethnic group [9, 10, 11]. Other studies have demonstrated a correlation between limited health literacy and an increase in preventable hospital visits and admissions exists [12, 13]. Patients with limited health literacy suffer from issues such as misunderstanding how to take a medication as directed and warnings on prescription labels [4]. Issues such as these, if addressed properly, have a better chance of being avoided if physicians implement methods to maximize patient comprehension and retention. By improving the health literacy of the public accordingly, we can maximize efficiency within a hospital by minimizing these preventable visits.

2. Methods of Improving Health Literacy

Patient compliance and adherence describe the degree to which patients correctly follow medical advice and recommendations from their physicians. Adherence has been shown to positively impact treatment outcomes [49]. Patient non-compliance poses a significant burden to a patient and his/her health, especially for those with chronic illnesses, undermining current medical care benefits [50]. Current research shows that health literacy can be used as a means of improving treatment adherence [51, 52, 53]. In one such study, patients with higher health literacies had a 14% higher rate of adherence than those with low health literacies [54]. Furthermore, patients that received interventions seeking to improve their health literacy had a 16% higher rate of adherence than those that did not receive any interventions [54]. The patient-doctor relationship is a key area of interest when seeking to increase compliance [55]. The health literacy-adherence relationship seems to be disease dependent, as demonstrated by higher compliance in patients with cardiovascular disease compared to other diseases [54]. The consequences of lifestyle and medication nonadherence in cardiovascular disease can be severe, and thus, patients may be more willing to adhere to their regimens with better understanding and proper education from physicians and medical resources [54].

a) Teach-Back Method

Physicians need to assess a patient's level of health literacy and address the patient in a manner that is appropriate to their level of understanding. Utilizing information-gathering questions such as "tell me what you already know about..." and "what else would you like to know about…" helps a physician assess patient comprehension and can help to establish a mutual agenda between the physician and patient. Communicating effectively with patients is important when ensuring patient safety, patient self-management, and efficient use of time [8]. Key strategies when communicating effectively include maintaining eye contact, slowing down, repeating main points, using plain, non-medical language, and encouraging patient participation [8]. The teach-back method is a commonly used practice by physicians in order to ensure that the information a physician relays to a patient is explained in a manner that the patient understands [8]. With this method, patients are asked to explain the information back to the physician in their own words, ensuring that the physician explained the concepts fully and in a manner that the patient can understand. If a patient cannot explain the information, then it is up to the physician to explain the concepts in another manner, which is more appropriate to the patient.

The teach-back method can be used to teach many concepts and techniques, and is appropriately also named the "show-me" method. Physicians may initiate by saying "I want to ensure that I did a good job explaining this, can you tell me how you would do what we discussed?" This helps avoid information overload and hones in to the information the physician feels is most important for the patient to retain. It's a method that can be used quite commonly in practice, even outside the medical field. This technique should be used after difficult concepts are explained. Some examples of using this method include prescribing an inhaler to a patient with asthma, advising an overweight patient with the proper foods to eat and avoid, and weighing the benefits and risks of a treatment plan. For example, when describing to a diabetic patient how to inject insulin, it may be beneficial to ask the patient to show you how they would inject the insulin. By doing so, you are dually confirming that the patient is able to complete the task and also fixing any errors in the technique. Patients are more satisfied with their physicians and retain more information about their illness when they are asked to restate what they are told [21]. One study showed that patients' retentions increased from 60.8% to 83.5% when the technique was used [21]. Another study demonstrated that utilizing the teach-back method with appointment scheduling may even be beneficial to patients. By having the patient repeat when their appointment is, patient compliance increased and the risk of missing an appointment decreased [41].

The teach-back method is extremely beneficial for many patients, including patients who have chronic illnesses who need to manage complex regimens and balance numerous appointments with various clinicians. These patients already have a lot of information regarding their health and thus, by asking them to repeat the information provided at an appointment, it ensures the physician adequately explained the relevant concepts. For instance, improved glycemic control among patients with diabetes mellitus has been observed when utilizing the teach-back method, regardless of the patient's literacy status [22]. To that effect, a physician should use the teach-back method with all patients, even if a physician feels that his/her patient has fully understood the information.

b) Improving Print Materials

Over 90 million Americans have limited health literacy and healthcare education materials need to be written simply for maximal patient comprehension. The National Institutes of Health and the American Medical Association recommend that patient resources be written at a 3rd to 7th grade level [63]. However, previous studies show that patient materials are more complex, written at a 7th to 9th grade level, some even at an 8th-12th grade level [61]. One such study showed that after analyzing patient education materials for those with chronic kidney disease, most materials were written at a 9th grade level, and only 5% were written at a 5th grade level [32]. Another study analyzed the literacy level of several different dental resources and found similar findings. Patient materials varied from a 3rd to 23rd grade level, with 41.7% of materials being written at a level below the average 7th to 9th grade level [33]. Many of these documents were written at or near a collegiate level. Another report demonstrated that most patient education materials from the American Academy of Orthopaedic Surgeons was disseminated at a level of 9.2, exceeding the average level [34]. This makes it clear that patient education materials are written at a level that is too complex for patients to adequately comprehend. By lowering the reading level that patient materials are compiled, patients may be better able to understand medical information circulated to them.

One possibility for lowering the reading level that resources are compiled may be to create a partnership between physicians and patients when constructing patient resources. Patients and families have many experiences and insight into the healthcare industry and may provide as a valuable resource in quality improvement and enhancing care. In creating a partnership between patients and medical personnel, resources would be created in a manner that is understandable and relevant for the average individual. This could decrease the amount of medical jargon that can be found within pamphlets, brochures, and other materials, increasing comprehension among patients [64].

c) Health Information on the Internet

Considering that over half of the Internet population use online materials as a resource when searching for health information, one possibility for improving healthcare materials is to focus efforts on online content. In regards to their health, the top three reasons individuals used the Internet was for communications (email), online communities (virtual support groups), and for medical information [15].

The third top reason individuals use the Internet is for healthcare information. Although this may greatly benefit patients by increasing their knowledge of various diseases, there are few guidelines and restrictions in place overseeing the quality of the information provided online as patients search for health information [19]. This puts individuals at risk of finding information that may be inaccurate and unreliable. Patients feel more in control as they gather as much information as they can, which helps to alleviate some of their concerns and fears. Individuals are constantly seeing and hearing different health messages on billboards on their drive to work, subway signs, television, and online. Even different physicians have varying ways of explaining concepts and thus, information may become misconstrued between providers, as seen with physicians as disclosing a dementia diagnosis. Variability was seen between providers in deciding whether to disclose a diagnosis, who to disclose a diagnosis to, and when to disclose a diagnosis of dementia [65]. Providing some form of oversight may minimize the amount of inconsistency between different mediums. This may be accomplished by utilizing a certification system, such as the Health on the Net (HON) code, that governs authorship, complementarity, confidentiality, attribution, justifiability, transparency, financial disclosure and advertising to ensure that health information provided on the Internet is consistent between sources [31].

By utilizing a certification system to assess the consistency between sources and a scale such as the LIDA scale to measure a site's validity, the information that patients seek can be improved to be accurate and relevant. The LIDA scale, consisting of 41 questions, is a tool used to measure the validity of a healthcare website [31]. The scale assess the quality of a resource based on the three domains: accessibility, reliability, and usability [31].

In order to reach a broad audience, healthcare websites need to be accessible to the public. This includes allowing the full text of a site to be both free to the public and compatible with the majority of browsers [31]. Few websites extend beyond English and Spanish, despite over 376 languages being used in the United States [43]. Disseminating healthcare information without other language options alienates the vast population of non-native American speakers. Thus, linguistic accessibility of online material is crucial for maximizing healthcare literacy. One study analyzed 122 health related websites and found that none of the websites fulfilled all of the Web accessibility requirements, including nonreliance on color alone, providing alternatives to auditory and visual content, ensuring user control over time-sensitvie changes, and clarifying natural language usage [44]. When measured with the LIDA scale, accessibility includes the validity of a HTML code, optimal alignment of text and images, and access restrictions [31]. Disparities in access to health information can lead to a lower use of preventive services, less knowledge of chronic disease management, and poorer overall health status [20]. As physicians suggest different resources for patients to utilize, they should ensure that patients are actually able to gain access to them. This includes identifying what resources the patient has readily available to them and providing resources within that medium. For example, if patients have Internet access, physicians may recommend specific websites for patients to gather additional information. However, if patients do not have Internet access, physicians need to provide the same information via another whether through brochures, pamphlets, or other print sources. Identifying patients' current access to healthcare reources is a critical step in improving health literacy.

In addition to accessing websites, patients with limited English proficiency (LEP) need to have access to additional resources to access patient information. When interacting with patients with LEP, such as deaf and Spanish speaking patients, further resources need to be utilized to fully improve quality of care. Increased accessibility and usability of interpreters and translators may be beneficial in this regard. For example, deaf patients enrolled in a primary care program that included full-time interpreters were more satisfied with physician communications and relayed improved preventive care outcomes [45]. Interventions such as using community health workers, health coaches, language interpreters, and language-concordant providers may prove to increase health literacy among LEP populations [46].

Usability referes to sources that are easy to use and provide the information that users are looking for. Agarwal et al., utilized the LIDA survey to interrogate the usability of three neurosurgical websites, and upon surveying them (AANS, Healthwise, and NINDS), it was determined that these sites were moderately usable [31]. This was based on grading criteria of consistency, clarity, functionality, and ability to engage [31]. Resources with a high degree of usability should utilize visual images and other multimedia resources. Thus, when presenting already complicated information, patients may grasp information better when provided non-textual media. Videos help break down complex material in a manner that is more readily understood. Furthermore, usable resources should take advantage of search and advanced search options, which are of great benefit to users [31]. Advanced search tools narrow the possible results when typing in key words and hone in on sources that are relaying specific information geared to the user's search criteria. Lastly, it may be beneficial to specifically highlight "Patient Education" tabs in order to de-clutter the information already present on a site [31].

One of the main concerns with usability is whether patients understand the information that is provided through a resource. With the current average American reading at an eighth grade level, health resources should be geared to an audience with a third to seventh grade reading level, so that they can be readily understood [47]. In doing so, a wider audience will be able to understand health information that is already complex. With increased understanding, patients can better ask their physicians appropriate questions and make informed decisions regarding their health. Compiling the material for an audience with lower literacy will not leave out information; rather it means that the material will be written in more plain language. If individuals with health literacy levels below the average reading level are still having difficulty grasping the material, further resources should be provided to increase comprehension and retention.

Another topic to consider is expanding the usability for individuals with disabilities. As individuals age, their health starts to decline. Many individuals have trouble seeing the small text presented on a webpage and would benefit from a large text option. Also to accommodate color-blind individuals, black and white formatting would increase usability for these users. These personalization features would help increase usability and continue to provide individuals with increased decision-making abilities.

With regards to reliability, citing sources helps to increase a site's transparency and thus, it's reputability [31]. By providing users the original source material, users can gain reliable information and further enables patients to make informed decisions regarding their health, as they are able to discuss material in detail with their healthcare providers [31].

d) Email Communications between Patients and Their Providers

Many patients are not able to ask all of the questions they may have during their appointment with their physician. This is potentially due to many reasons such as simply forgetting or after given some time to process the information a physician provided, further questions arise. Patients may not know what questions they should be asking based on their diagnosis. Information-gathering questions help assess why a patient is present and what a patient wants out of a visit. A study showed that 87% of patients wanted all of the information possible about their diagnosis and 54% were not satisfied with the information provided by their healthcare providers [17, 18]. Thus, patients may seek the Internet for additional information regarding their illness or disease. With email communications being the primary reason for Internet use, email communications could help to facilitate the patient-physician relationship due to the ability to ask questions as they arise and even by minimizing unnecessary visits [16]. Furthermore, email communications provide an added benefit over telephone communications or in-office visits with a physician, as physicians have flexibility upon responding. Secure email communications may increase the efficacy of care by replacing some outpatient visits [42]. Kaiser Permanente followed 35,423 patients and found that the top five reasons that patients email their physicians are to discuss a change in health condition, lab results, a new condition, drug dosages, or a new drug [42]. In this study, patients with hypertension and diabetes were followed, and patients that used email to communicate with their physicians were found to have a statistically significant increase in effectiveness of care [42]. HbA1c levels had a difference of 11.1 on the HEDIS Effectiveness of Care scale between patients that utilized email to communicate with their physicians and those that did not utilize email, with patients that utilized email communications having lower HbA1c levels [42]. Furthermore, increases in cholesterol and blood pressure control were found to be improved 2.0-6.5% in patients utilizing email for physician communications [42]. By effectively leveraging email communications with patients, healthcare providers can improve the efficacy of healthcare delivery.

e) Health Media Coverage

Health information is not limited to the Internet; another medium that affects a large population is mass news media. The Bureau of Labor Statistics reported that in 2014, the average American above the age of 15 watched an average of 2.8 hours of T.V. daily [23].

Health news coverage influences health knowledge and behaviors. For example, after Katie Couric's segment on NBC's Today Show in 2000 demonstrating the importance of having a colonoscopy, colonoscopies increased by 27% [24]. Over ¾ of Americans reported on acting on the health information presented from mass media [25, 26]. However, this poses a large risk, as the average median airtime for a health story is 33 seconds [27]. Mass media generally covers new health stories or uncommon events such as the West Nile Virus, which gained the media's attention in 2002 [27]. Most stories reported the number of infected people and deaths within a specific community, but failed to relay the relatively low incidence compared to other diseases [27]. Only 18% of stories discussing the West Nile Virus discussed prevention strategies in avoiding mosquitos or what to do if bitten by a mosquito [27]. By discussing prevention strategies, news outlets can assuage fears within the public and minimize the number of individuals seeking medical attention after being bitten by a mosquito [27]. Healthcare professionals should have an input into which stories are being aired and assist in providing proper prevention techniques. Sometimes news outlets focus on eye-catching stories, rather than the stories pertinent to the public. For example, the majority of stories discussing cancer involve sex-specific cancers, such as breast cancer and cervical cancer, over lung cancer, which is the leading cause of cancer-mortality [27]. Another issue that is extremely grave is reporting on information that is inaccurate or oversimplified. One health story reported that lemon juice might be a substitute for costly HIV medications [27]. Another story displayed a headline stating "breast self-examinations may be a waste of time" [27]. This type of information is not only extremely misleading, but will negatively affect patients, who choose to act on this information.

There is no credential requirement needed to report on health information. Just as meteorologists have further training to report on the weather, there should be some form of specialized training when reporting health information [27]. This will increase accuracy of information, validity, and credibility of the source.

f) Patient Portals

Patient portal adoption has rapidly increased over the last few decades [58]. Patient portals are online tools that provide patients with 24/7 access to portions of their health records, as well as interactions with healthcare systems and providers [58]. These resources allow patients to be engaged with their health, increase their self-efficacy, and improve the quality of care [58]. However, typically, a medically illiterate population is less likely to use patient portals, preferring information to be reported in person or on the phone [60, 61]. One study reported an association between health literacy and registration for portal use, such that patients with higher health literacies were more likely to be registered for a patient portal than patients with lower literacies [58]. Promoting patient portal adoption among healthcare providers and use may help to increase patient confidence, patient satisfaction, and clinical outcomes [58].

3. Impact of Improving Health Literacy

Highly health literate patients are more likely to understand more about their personal health condition. Patients with low health literacy are at risk for not comprehending what their physician is instructing them to do and thus, may not understand the full extent of their illness and treatment regimen. For example, one study compared patient literacy level with knowledge of their condition in a population of patients with hypertension and diabetes [35]. Almost half of the patients had limited health literacy and thus, had significantly less knowledge of the disease and self-management practices. One-third of the patients did not know that losing weight reduces blood pressure levels and almost two-thirds did not know that exercise reduces blood pressure, despite having attended formal education classes regarding their illnesses [35]. This shows that a gap is present within current educational strategies, as the majority of the information does not effectively reach those with poor levels of literacy.

With less knowledge their own illnesses, patients cannot adequately practice successful self-management. Greater health literacy allows one to manage medications, avoid triggers, and monitor symptoms [36]. Patients with lower health literacy and chronic comorbidities such as asthma are at risk for having negative outcomes. Asthma patients with low health literacy have been shown to have more negative outcomes such as worse asthma-related quality of life, worse physical function, and more emergency department use over a period of 2 years, compared to their more health literate counterparts [36]. These outcomes may be due to many factors, such as patients utilizing their inhalers incorrectly and inadequate knowledge of what to do during an asthma attack [36]. Another analysis in that report demonstrated that patients with adequate health literacy, 89% considered asthma attacks harmful, whereas 66% of lower health literate patients were less likely to consider these attacks harmful [36]. This poses as a threat to patient outcomes, as patients may not recognize potentially dangerous disease sequelae and practice proper preventative regimens.

Furthermore, as treatment modalities improve and become more complicated, patients must take on more duties than they did in the past. For example, patients with congestive heart failure were prescribed digoxin and diuretics in the past, while today's patients take loop diuretics, beta blockers, angiotensin converting enzyme inhibitors, spironolactone, and digoxin [4]. In addition to these medications, these patients were simply instructed to decrease their physical activity in the past, whereas now, patients are asked to eat low sodium diets, weigh themselves daily, report any weight gains to their physicians, and to participate in structured exercise [4]. Patients need to take many extra steps to adequately take care of themselves as the complexity of medical care increases. However, studies show that 40-80% of the medical information that patients receive is forgotten immediately and nearly half of the information that is remembered is inaccurate [7, 8].

Poor health literacy nationwide has been shown to increase national healthcare spending and is estimated to cost around $1.6 to $3.6 trillion [30]. Patients with lower health literacy generated significantly higher annual mean total healthcare charges [40]. Low-level readers generated $10,688 whereas high-level readers generated $2,891 total healthcare charges annually [40]. These differences were mainly accounted for by inpatient charges, $7,038 vs. $824, for low-level readers and high-level readers, respectively [40]. This is supported by key findings in which lower literacy is associated with poorer health status, increased hospitalization, and emergency department visits [40]. Furthermore, research has shown that low income and traditionally underserved populations are at risk for lower health literacy [56, 57]. Interestingly, interventions aiming at improving health literacy were more effective among lower income patients than in patients with higher incomes [54].

Another impact of low health literacy among patients is increased mortality. For instance, kidney disease is the 9th leading cause of death in the United States [37]. Many patients with kidney disease must undergo routine dialysis, which is a very time-consuming task, generally lasting 4 hours per treatment for three times a week [37]. Patients who have a high level of medical literacy may have improved health via increased general knowledge about their illness, improved communication between providers, and greater self-efficacy in care related to kidney disease [37]. Patients with lower health literacy are at risk for failing to adhere to medications and dialysis schedules. Kidney disease patients with low health literacy have been shown to understand less about their health condition, which may predispose them to missing symptomology or other risk factors for disease progression and increased mortality [37].

Both physical and mental health are affected by low health literacy. Patients with low health literacy tend to display more depressive symptoms. The Centers for Epidemiologic Studies-Depression (CES-D) scores measure depressive symptoms. Scores range from 0-60 and a higher CES-D score indicates a higher level of distress, with a score greater or equal to 16 indicating a clinically significant level of distress [38]. When analyzing patients struggling with addiction, it was found that patients with low health literacy were 3 times more likely to have depression, with a mean CES-D score of 26.7 [38]. One of the factors that may contribute to these higher levels of depression may be the shame felt by patients with low medical literacy [38]. Many patients may not admit their difficulty reading due to feeling shameful. Of patients that have low functional health literacy, 67.2% had not told their spouses that they had difficulty reading and understanding and 19% had never disclosed their difficulty to anyone [39]. Given these statistics, physicians may be overestimating patient comprehension, given the substantial portion of patients that do not disclose their misunderstanding.

Health literacy in the pediatric population presents another challenging topic. Parents tend to take charge of a child's health regimen and thus, children are left with minimal knowledge of their health and health regimen [28]. In a survey conducted to see if children, aged 6-18, had medical knowledge regarding their cancer medications, they were asked questions such as: what are your medications? How do they work? How do you take them? Why do you take them? [28] These children had limited knowledge on their medications, knowing the color of their medications and generally when they take the medications, but did not understand the purpose of taking the medication and how it worked inside the body [28]. Furthermore, 73% of these patients stated that the physicians directed the conversation to the parent and 64% were not even in the room during the visit [28]. Of course some of this can be attributed to a child's minimal speaking capabilities or a parent's sense of ease in assisting their child. However, this may also be attributed to a child's lower health literacy or a lack of teaching provided from a physician. By encouraging children at a young age to participate in the conversation, they gain self-confidence and a feeling of importance [29]. 81% of children in this study stated that they want to be involved in their medications and were eager to learn more [29]. As health literacy is a skill that develops over time and is shaped by medical exposure, health literacy may be improved by starting earlier. Other measures may be considered such as starting health initiatives within educational settings earlier. This could increase interaction with and general knowledge of the healthcare setting at an earlier age.

Many methods for improving healthcare literacy were discussed in this chapter and they must be readily accepted and applied by healthcare providers for efficacious reform. A significant challenge is identifying patients who would most readily benefit from these mehtodologies. Patients may actually hide their level of literacy from their provider, due to a sense of shame in lacking health knowledge, making it difficult for physicians to accurately assess a patient's level of understanding. To that effect, utilizing methods like the teach-back method and information-gathering questions, are extremely important in bridging the gap between a physician and patient. By understanding the level the patient is at in understanding the information provided, physicians will be able to personalize the conversation, gearing it towards a patient's level of understanding. With constant encouragement from the right sources, such as physicians, patients will feel more empowered and encouraged to play an active role with their health, leading to better health outcomes [48].

REFERENCES

[1] U.S. Department of Health and Human Services, O.o.D.P.a.H.S., *National Action Plan to Improve Health Literacy.* 2010.

[2] Agarwal, N., et al., Educational Resources "Over the Head" of Neurosurgical Patients: The Economic Impact of Inadequate Health Literacy. *World Neurosurg*, 2015. **84**(5): p. 1223-6.

[3] Walsh, T.M. and T.A. Volsko, Readability assessment of Internet-based consumer health information. *Respir Care,* 2008. **53**(10): p. 1310-5.

[4] Weiss, B.D., *{Kissel, 2007 #67}*. 2007, Chicago, IL: AMA Foundation.

[5] Davis TC, Dolan NC, Ferreira MR, Tomori C, Green KW, Sipler AM, Bennett CL. The role of inadequate health literacy skills in colorectal cancer screening. *Cancer Invest.* 2001;19:193-200.

[6] Davis TC, Arnold C, Berkel HJ, Nandy I, Jackson RH, Glass J. Knowledge and attitude on screening mammography among low-literate, low-income women. *Cancer.* 1996;78:1912-1920.

[7] Kutner M, Greenberg E, Jin Y, Paulsen C. The Health Literacy of America's Adults: Results from the 2003 National Assessment of Adult Literacy. US Department of Education. National Center for Education Statistics, 2006. *NCES Publication* No. 2006-483.

[8] DeWalt DA, Berkman ND, Sheridan S, et al., Literacy and health outcomes: a systematic review of the literature. *J Gen Intern Med.* 2004;19(12):1228-39.

[9] Weiss BD, Hart G, McGee D, D'Estelle S. Health status of illiterate adults: relation between literacy and health status among persons with low literacy skills. *J Am Board Fam Pract.* 1992;5:257-264.

[10] Baker D, Parker R, Williams MV, Clark WS, Nurss J. The relationship of patient reading ability to selfreported health and use of health services. *Am J Public Health.* 1997;87:1027-1030.

[11] Sudore RL, Yaffe K, Satterfield S, Harris TB, et al., Limited literacy and mortality in the elderly: the health, aging, and body composition study. *J Gen Intern Med.* 2006;21:806-812.

[12] Nielsen-Bohlman, L., Panzer, A. M. and Kindig, D. A. (Eds.). (2004). *Health literacy: A prescription to end confusion*. Washington, DC: National Academies Press.

[13] Berkman, N. D., DeWalt, D. A., Pignone, M. P., Sheridan, S. L., Lohr, K. N., Lux, L., et al., (2004). *Literacy and health outcomes* (AHRQ Publication No. 04-E007-2). Rockville, MD: Agency for Healthcare Research and Quality.

[14] Pew Internet and American Life Project. *The Social Life of Health* Information. 2011. http://pewInternet.org/~/media//Files/Reports/2011/ PIP_Social_Life_of_Health_Info.pdf. Accessed February 28, 2012.

[15] Eysenbach, G: The Impact of the Internet on Cancer Outcomes. *CA: A Cancer Journal for Clinicians*. 2003; 53:356-371.

[16] Mechanic D. How should hamsters run? Some observations about sufficient patient time in primary care. *BMJ* 2001;323:266–268.

[17] Jenkins V, Fallowfield L, Saul J. Information needs of patients with cancer: results from a large study in UK cancer centres. *Br J Cancer* 2001; 84:48–51.

[18] Chen X, Siu LL. Impact of the media and the Internet on oncology: survey of cancer patients and oncologists in Canada. *J Clin Oncol* 2001; 19:4291–4297.

[19] D'Alessandro DM, Kingsley P, Johnson-West J: The readability of pediatric patient education materials on the World Wide Web. *Arch Pediatr Adolesc Med* 155:807-812, 2001.

[20] Berkman ND, DeWalt DA, Pignone MP, et al., Literacy and health outcomes: Summary [Internet]. Rockville, MD: Agency for Healthcare Research and Quality; 2004 Jan. 8 p. (AHRQ publication; no. 04-E007-1); (Evidence report/technology assessment; no. 87).

[21] Bertakis K. The communication of information from physician to patient: a method for increasing patient retention and satisfaction. *J Fam Prac* 1977;5(2):217-222.

[22] Schillinger D, Piette J, Grumbach K, Wang F, Wilson C, Daher C, Leong-Grotz K, Castro C, Bindman AB. Closing the loop: physician communication with diabetic patients who have low health literacy. *Arch Intern Med.* 2003;163:83-90.

[23] "American Time Use Survey Summary." *U.S. Bureau of Labor Statistics*. U.S. Bureau of Labor Statistics, 24 June 2015.

[24] Cram P, Fendrick AM, Inadomi J, Cowen ME, Carpenter D, Vijan S. The impact of a celebrity promotional campaign on the use of colon cancer screening: the Katie Couric effect. *Arch Intern Med.* 2003;163:1601-1605.

[25] National Health Council. 21st Century House Call: The Link between Medicine and the Media. Washington, DC: National Health Council; December 1997.

[26] National Health Council. Americans Talk About Science and Medical News. Washington, DC: National Health Council; December 1997.

[27] Pribble, JM, Goldstein KM, Fowler EF, Greenberg MJ, Noel SK, Howell JD. Medical News for the Public to Use? What's on Local TV News? *The American Journal of Managed Care*. 2006; 12: 170-176.

[28] MacDonald T, MacDonald D, Crooks B, Collicott C. What do children with cancer know about their medications? Pharmacy Practice (Internet) 2011 Oct-Dec;9(4):207-212.

[29] Abrams MA, Klass P, Dreyer BP. Health Literacy and Children: Introduction. *Pediatrics*. 2009;124(suppl 3):S262-S264.

[30] Vernon, J. A., Trujillo, A., Rosenbaum, S. and DeBuono, B. (2007). Low health literacy: Implications for national policy.

[31] Agarwal, N., et al., Accessibility, Reliability, and Usability of Neurosurgical Resources. *Journal of Neurosurgery*, 2015.

[32] Morony, S., et al., Readability of Written Materials for CKD Patients: A Systematic Review. *Am J Kidney Dis*, 2015. **65**(6): p. 842-50.

[33] Alexander, R.E., *Readability of published dental educational materials. J Am Dent Assoc*, 2000. **131**(7): p. 937-42.

[34] Eltorai, A.E., et al., Most American Academy of Orthopaedic Surgeons' online patient education material exceeds average patient reading level. *Clin Orthop Relat Res*, 2015. **473**(4): p. 1181-6.

[35] Williams, M.V., et al., Relationship of functional health literacy to patients' knowledge of their chronic disease. A study of patients with hypertension and diabetes. *Arch Intern Med*, 1998. **158**(2): p. 166-72.

[36] Mancuso, C.A. and M. Rincon, Impact of health literacy on longitudinal asthma outcomes. *J Gen Intern Med*, 2006. **21**(8): p. 813-7.

[37] Cavanaugh, K.L., et al., Low health literacy associates with increased mortality in ESRD. *J Am Soc Nephrol*, 2010. **21**(11): p. 1979-85.

[38] Lincoln, A., et al., Impact of health literacy on depressive symptoms and mental health-related: quality of life among adults with addiction. *J Gen Intern Med, 2006*. **21**(8): p. 818-22.

[39] Parikh, N.S., et al., Shame and health literacy: the unspoken connection. *Patient Educ Couns,* 1996. **27**(1): p. 33-9.

[40] Weiss, B.D. and R. Palmer, Relationship between healthcare costs and very low literacy skills in a medically needy and indigent Medicaid population. *J Am Board Fam Pract*, 2004. **17**(1): p. 44-7.

[41] Schillinger, D., et al., *Association of health literacy with diabetes outcomes. JAMA,* 2002. **288**(4): p. 475-82.

[42] Zhou, Y.Y., et al., Improved quality at Kaiser Permanente through e-mail between physicians and patients. *Health Aff (Millwood),* 2010. **29**(7): p. 1370-5.

[43] Schillinger, D., et al., Functional health literacy and the quality of physician-patient communication among diabetes patients. *Patient Educ Couns,* 2004. **52**(3): p. 315-23.
[44] Zeng, X. and B. Parmanto, Evaluation of web accessibility of consumer health information websites. *AMIA Annu Symp Proc*, 2003: p. 743-7.
[45] MacKinney, T.G., et al., Improvements in preventive care and communication for deaf patients: results of a novel primary healthcare program. *J Gen Intern Med*, 1995. **10**(3): p. 133-7.
[46] McKee, M.M. and M.K. Paasche-Orlow, Health literacy and the disenfranchised: the importance of collaboration between limited English proficiency and health literacy researchers. *J Health Commun*, 2012. **17** Suppl **3**: p. 7-12.
[47] Walsh, T.M. and T.A. Volsko, Readability assessment of Internet-based consumer health information. *Respir Care*, 2008. **53**(10): p. 1310-5.
[48] Agarwal, N., et al., A comparative analysis of the quality of patient education materials from medical specialties. *JAMA Internal Medicine*, 2013. **173**(13): p. 1257-1259.
[49] Modi, A.C. and A.L. Quittner, Barriers to treatment adherence for children with cystic fibrosis and asthma: what gets in the way? *J Pediatr Psychol*, 2006. **31**(8): p. 846-58.
[50] Martin, L.R., et al., The challenge of patient adherence. *Ther Clin Risk Manag,* 2005. **1**(3): p. 189-99.
[51] Wolf, M.S., et al., Literacy, self-efficacy, and HIV medication adherence. *Patient Educ Couns,* 2007. **65**(2): p. 253-60.
[52] Zhang, N.J., A. Terry, and C.A. McHorney, Impact of health literacy on medication adherence: a systematic review and meta-analysis. *Ann Pharmacother,* 2014. **48**(6): p. 741-51.
[53] Baker, D.W., The meaning and the measure of health literacy. *J Gen Intern Med*, 2006. **21**(8): p. 878-83.
[54] Miller, T.A., Health literacy and adherence to medical treatment in chronic and acute illness: A meta-analysis. *Patient Educ Couns*, 2016. **99**(7): p. 1079-86.
[55] Donovan, J.L., Patient decision making. The missing ingredient in compliance research. *Int J Technol Assess Healthcare*, 1995. **11**(3): p. 443-55.
[56] Paasche-Orlow, M.K., et al., Health literacy, antiretroviral adherence, and HIV-RNA suppression: a longitudinal perspective. *J Gen Intern Med,* 2006. **21**(8): p. 835-40.

[57] Sudore, R.L., et al., Use of a modified informed consent process among vulnerable patients: a descriptive study. *J Gen Intern Med*, 2006. **21**(8): p. 867-73.
[58] Davis, S.E., et al., Health Literacy, Education Levels, and Patient Portal Usage During Hospitalizations. *AMIA Annu Symp Proc*, 2015. **2015**: p. 1871-80.
[59] Morris, N.S., et al., Prevalence of limited health literacy and compensatory strategies used by hospitalized patients. *Nurs Res*, 2011. **60**(5): p. 361-6.
[60] Sarkar, U., et al., Social disparities in Internet patient portal use in diabetes: evidence that the digital divide extends beyond access. *J Am Med Inform Assoc*, 2011. **18**(3): p. 318-21.
[61] Sarkar, U., et al., Preferences for self-management support: findings from a survey of diabetes patients in safety-net health systems. *Patient Educ Couns,* 2008. **70**(1): p. 102-10.
[62] in *Health Literacy: A Prescription to End Confusion*, L. Nielsen-Bohlman, A.M. Panzer, and D.A. Kindig, Editors. 2004: Washington (DC).
[63] Kirsch IS, Jungeblut A, Jenkins L, Kolstad A. Adult Literacy in America: A First Look at the Results of the National Adult Literacy Survey. *Natl Cent Educ Stat*. 2002:178.
[64] Johnson, B., et al., Partnering with Patients and Families to Design a Patient and Family-Centered Healthcare System. 2008.
[65] Kissel, E.C. and B.D. Carpenter, It's all in the details: physician variability in disclosing a dementia diagnosis. *Aging Ment Health*, 2007. **11**(3): p. 273-80.

In: The Evolution of Health Literacy
Editors: N. Agarwal et al.
ISBN: 978-1-53610-602-2

Chapter 6

Socioeconomic Considerations: Economic Impact of Health Literacy

Prateek Agarwal*[1], *Divyansh Agarwal*[1], *Tejas Karnati*[2], *Tekchand Ramchand*[3], *MD* and *Carl Kraus*[4], *MD

[1]Perelman School of Medicine, University of Pennsylvania, Philadelphia, PA, US
[2]University of Pittsburgh School of Medicine, Pittsburgh, PA, US
[3]Department of Radiology, Yale University, New Haven, CT, US
[4]Department of Radiology, Columbia University, New York, NY, US

Abstract

In this chapter, we review the literature examining the socioeconomic considerations of health literacy. We focus on the overall economic impact and epidemiology of health literacy as well as how socioeconomic disparities in health literacy may lead to inferior health outcomes.

We determined that there is some evidence to suggest that low health literacy amongst patients with Medicare and consumer-driven health insurance is associated with increased health costs. From a health system perspective, some estimates of the annual excess cost of low health literacy range between 106 billion United States dollars (USD) and 238 billion USD. Epidemiological studies have shown that only 12% of

American adults have proficient health literacy, with adults over 65 having the lowest levels of health literacy.

Furthermore, minority race, less education, and lower income have been independently correlated with lower levels of health literacy. With regards to socioeconomic disparities, low health literacy has been demonstrated to result in poor health outcomes in disadvantaged or vulnerable populations. An extensive review of the literature in this chapter facilitates a clearer understanding of how the socioeconomic aspects of low health literacy negatively impact our society from both socioeconomic and health equity perspectives.

Economic Cost

Although the literature contains substantial evidence of the association between low health literacy levels and poor health outcomes [16], quantitative data on the *economic* impact of low health literacy is scarce. Many of the studies examine the excess cost within subsets of Medicare and Medicaid patient populations rather than estimating the excess cost to large or nationwide health systems. In this section, we review literature on the economic impact of low health literacy and report purposed aggregate unnecessary costs arising from low health literacy in the United States and other nations.

Medicaid, Medicare, and Consumer-Driven Health Insurance Patients

A subset of studies in the literature examines the economic impact of low health literacy in patients enrolled in Medicaid, Medicare, and consumer-driven health insurance plans (CDHPs). CDHPs are plans that combine high-deductible medical insurance with financial accounts and are offered by many health insurers such as Blue Cross Blue Shield, Aetna, Kaiser, Humana, etc. With regards to patients enrolled in Medicaid, Weiss and Palmer examined the association between literacy skills in English or Spanish and total annual healthcare charges. After adjusting for demographic variables, annual healthcare charges were found to be 10,688 USD for patients at or below a third-grade reading level, but only 2,981 USD for patients at or above a fourth-grade reading level ($p = 0.025$). It should be noted that the Weiss and Palmer study included only 74 patients, which the authors acknowledged to be a small sample size [1].

In a larger study of 3,260 patients enrolled in Medicare managed plans, Howard et al. investigated whether low health literacy increases medical care use and associated costs. The authors employed the Short Test of Functional Health Literacy in Adults (STOFHLA) to measure health literacy and adjusted for various potentially confounding demographic variables and comorbidities in a regression model. The measured outcomes included emergency room costs, inpatient costs, and total costs. The authors found that low health literacy was associated with a 108 USD increase in emergency room costs and that such a relationship was statistically significant. While they also found that low health literacy was associated with a 1,551 USD increase in total costs and a 1,543 USD increase in inpatient costs, these differences did not reach statistical significance [2].

A more recent and larger study of 4,130 patients enrolled in consumer-driven health insurance plans utilized a series of three questions to measure health literacy. In this study, Hardie et al. employed regression analysis to determine the effect of health literacy on healthcare spending while controlling for demographics and comorbidities. The authors found that lower health literacy scores on these three questions and the sum of the scores were associated with increased total healthcare spending, with increased emergency department and inpatient admission spending contributing to the bulk of the increase [3].

The three aforementioned studies all concluded that low health literacy had a substantial economic impact due to increases in healthcare expenditures for groups of patients enrolled in Medicaid, Medicare, and CDHPs.

Effect of Caregiver Literacy

The vast majority of studies that have investigated the economic impact of low health literacy focus on the health literacy skills of patients. However not all patient populations make their own health decisions; pediatric patients, for example, rely on caregivers to make such decisions. Hence the health literacy skills of caregivers have the potential to drive healthcare costs. To the best of our knowledge, there is only a single published study that examines caregiver health literacy and its relationship to healthcare cost: a cross-sectional study of caregiver-child pairs from a sample of children aged 12 months to 12 years in a pediatric emergency department of an urban, public hospital. Sanders et. al.

used the STOFHLA in English or Spanish to measure health literacy and assessed cost of child healthcare from Medicaid billing records. The STOFHLA has been well validated against other measures of literacy and reading ability according to the authors.

In regression models that controlled for demographics and special healthcare needs, the authors found no differences in healthcare cost between children with caregivers who had low health literacy and children with caregivers who had proficient health literacy (out of a total possible score of 36 on the STOFHLA, adults with a score < 17 were considered to have inadequate health literacy, while those with a score of 17 to 22 were considered to have marginal health literacy and those with a score ≥ 23 were considered to have proficient health literacy) [4]. This finding suggests that the health literacy skills of patients are more relevant for healthcare costs than the health literacy skills of caregivers, though it is important to note that the generalizability of this study is limited given its highly specific focus on caregivers of an inner city pediatric population. Future studies could explore the impact of health literacy on costs in elderly populations that are reliant on health choices dictated by caregivers.

Health System Effects

The aforementioned studies involved small groups of patients, but we are ultimately interested in the effects of low health literacy on entire health systems in terms of aggregate excess healthcare costs. A more recent study conducted by Haun et. al. explored this issue using data from the Veterans Health Administration on 92,749 patients.

In a generalized linear model that adjusted for demographics and other potential cofounding factors, the authors found that over a three-year period, inadequate and marginal health literacy were respectively associated with a 31,581 USD and 23,508 USD increase in cost per patient when compared to adequate health literacy. Overall, the authors calculated the excess healthcare cost over the three-year period due to marginal and inadequate health literacy to be 143 million USD [5].

Other studies have attempted to estimate the excess costs due to low health literacy for the entire United States health system and population. In a study by Friedland that used literacy data from the 1992 National Adult Literacy Survey and cost data from the 1993 Survey of Income and Program Participation, the additional cost to the United States healthcare system resulting from low health literacy was determined to be 69 billion USD. However, it should be noted that this survey did not include a dedicated assessment of health literacy [6]. More recently, Vernon et al. updated Friedland's estimate by adding data from the 2003 National Assessment of Adult Literacy survey (which directly assessed health literacy) and current healthcare expenditure data from the Medical Expenditure Panel Survey. Their report estimated the annual excess cost of the low health literacy to be between 106 billion USD and 238 billion USD [7, 8].

Using a standard social discount rate (a common measure applied to any statistical model when computing the value of funds spent on social projects), Vernon et al. estimated the present-day excess cost of low health literacy to be between 1.6 trillion USD and 3.6 trillion USD [7]. Such national cost estimates for entire health systems are sparse outside of the United States, although Spycher et al. did report an additional cost of 1.5 billion Swiss franc (CHF) due to low health literacy in Switzerland [9].

EPIDEMIOLOGY

Before discussing the relationship of socioeconomic status and health literacy with health outcomes, it is important to address the epidemiology of health literacy.Within the literature, the most reliable source of information on the epidemiology of health literacy comes from the United States Department of Education 2003 National Assessment of Adult Literacy, which contained a dedicated health literacy assessment component [10]. In this section, we describe the variable degrees of health literacy amongst seven different parameters: the total population, gender, race and ethnicity, native language, age, education level, and income.

Total Population

Amongst the total population, 12 percent of adults had proficient health literacy, 53 percent had intermediate health literacy, 22 percent had basic health literacy, and 14 percent had below basic health literacy [10]. A separate meta-analysis of 85 studies with 31,129 subjects reported low health literacy to be 26% and marginal health literacy to be 20% [11].

Gender

For women, the average health literacy score was 6 points higher than the average score for men. More men had below basic healthy literacy than women by 4 percentage points, and more women had intermediate health literacy by 4 percentage points. However, there were no significant differences between men and women with regards to proficient or basic health literacy [10], and a separate meta-analysis found no association between the prevalence of low health literacy and gender [11].

Age

Adults 65 years and older had the lowest average health literacy scores, while adults between the ages of 25 and 39 had the highest average scores. Perhaps most strikingly, only 38 percent of adults 65 and older had intermediate health literacy, while all other age groups had between 53 and 58 percent with intermediate health literacy. In addition, significantly more adults 65 and older had basic and below basic health literacy than all other age groups [10]. A separate meta-analysis validated the association between the prevalence of low health literacy and age [11].

Race and Ethnicity

With regards to average health literacy score, Hispanic adults had the lowest score of all racial/ethnic groups, and White and Asian/Pacific Islander adults had higher scores than Black, Hispanic, American Indian/Alaska Native, and Multiracial adults. More specifically, White and Asian/Pacific Islander adults had more proficient health literacy than other ethnic/racial groups, while Black and Hispanic adults had more basic and below basic health literacy than other ethnic/racial groups. For intermediate healthy literacy, the adult population was composed of 58 percent White, 52 percent Asian/Pacific Islander, 59 percent Multiracial, 41 percent Black, and 31 percent Hispanic adults [10]. A separate meta-analysis confirmed these findings, noting that black adults had the highest prevalence of low health literacy [11].

Native Language

As might be expected, participants who spoke English as their native language before starting school had higher average health literacy scores than those who spoke a native language other than English. On the other hand, participants who spoke only Spanish before school had the lowest average health literacy scores. Participants who spoke English and another language before starting school had an intermediate level mean health literacy score [10].

Education

As also might be expected, adults who had not attended or completed high school had the lowest average health literacy scores, and scores increased progressively with each additional higher level of education. Similarly, adults who had not attended or completed high school had the highest percentage of below basic health literacy among all other education groups and the second-to-lowest percentage of proficient health literacy. Adults who had taken some graduate classes, completed a graduate degree, or graduated from a 4-year college had the highest levels of proficient health literacy [10]. Again, a meta-analysis confirmed the association between low health literacy and level of education [11].

Income

Those adults living below the poverty level, at the poverty level, or up to 125 percent of the poverty level had a significantly lower average health literacy score than higher-income adults. The average health literacy scores of these adults corresponded to a basic level, whereas the average health literacy scores of adults living above 17 percent of the poverty level corresponded to an intermediate level [10].

SOCIOECONOMIC STATUS, HEALTH LITERACY, AND HEALTH OUTCOMES

Socioeconomic status is a composite measure of an individuals' income, education and occupation. Multiple studies have demonstrated that lower socioeconomic status is associated with increased poor health outcomes [12-15]. One posited theory to explain this association argues that individuals from lower socioeconomic status demonstrate higher "health risk" behavior, such as cigarette smoking and sedentary lifestyle [16], therefore leading to higher mortality. However, in this section we present studies that suggest differences in health outcomes among those of lower socioeconomic status is influenced independently by factors such as income and health literacy.

In a study conducted by Lantz et al., authors examined the influence of income and education on mortality rates among individuals of differing risk behaviors (e.g., smoking) and demographics such as age, race, urbanicity, sex. They found that individuals with lower income and education levels, while controlling for risk behaviors and demographic differences, had higher mortality rates. Hence, the authors concluded that higher mortality among individuals with lower socioeconomic standing cannot be purely attributed to increased "risk behaviors". Health literacy has been shown to significantly influence health outcomes in both the pediatric and adult populations [17]. Additionally, low caregiver literacy has been associated with poor preventive care behaviors [17]. For instance, in a study examining the relationship between health literacy and child health, it was found that at least a third of the young adults had low health literacy. After adjusting for socioeconomic status, adults with low health literacy were 1.2 to 4 times more likely to exhibit negative health behaviors that affected child health. Adolescents with low health literacy were at least twice as likely to exhibit aggressive or antisocial behavior, and chronically ill children who had caregivers with low health literacy were twice as likely to use more health services [17].

In a low-income population with a particular disease or disorder, the finding that health literacy mediates the relationship between education and health outcomes has important implications for both education and health policy. For example, Schillinger et al. [18] sought to determine whether health literacy mediated the relationship between education and glycemic control among diabetes patients. The study concluded that educational attainment was associated with better glycemic control, particularly when comparing two lower strata of education (less than high school graduate level versus high school graduate level). The differences observed were both statistically and clinically significant. Results such as these and other similar studies [19-22] suggest that health literacy, at least in part, mediates the relationship between education and glycemic control in a population of low-income patients with diabetes. A possible mechanism underlying this observation is that individuals with inadequate literacy have been demonstrated to have clinically significant problems with communication, both written and oral [23, 24].

There is increasing evidence in the medical literature to indicate that increasing the health literacy of patients could be one part of a multifaceted strategy to address non-adherence to prescription medications [25]. A meta-analysis found higher health literacy levels to be associated with better medication adherence across 6 diseases and 35 samples [26]. It has been speculated that health literacy may influence a patient's medication beliefs, which can significantly influence medication adherence. Additional links have been examined between health literacy and race disparities in HIV-medication adherence. Though Osborn et al. found that African-American patients had a two-fold greater likelihood of being non-adherent to their anti-retroviral regimens, the correlation with race was weakened when the confounding variable of health literacy was taken into account [27].

Overall, limited health literacy presents a wide-reaching barrier to accomplishing desirable health outcomes. The link between health literacy, socioeconomic disparities, and health outcomes has important policy implications because one can develop better communication strategies and focus implementation of those strategies in populations with the greatest need. Instructional and design improvements can contribute to vastly reducing disparities [28-30]. Devoting resources to educational strategies that are both culturally sensitive as well as appropriate for lower-literacy audiences may greatly benefit patients.

REFERENCES

[1] Weiss B. D., Palmer R. Relationship between healthcare costs and very low literacy skills in a medically needy and indigent Medicaid population. *J. Am. Board Fam. Pract.,* 2004; 17(1):44-47.

[2] Howard D. H., Gazmararian J., Parker R. M. The impact of low health literacy on the medical costs of Medicare managed care enrollees. *Am. J. Med.,* 2005; 118(4):371-377.

[3] Hardie N. A., Kyanko K., Busch S., Losasso A. T., Levin R. A. Health literacy and healthcare spending and utilization in a consumer-driven health plan. *J. Health Commun.,* 2011; 16 Suppl. 3:308-321.
[4] Sanders L. M., Thompson V. T., Wilkinson J. D. Caregiver health literacy and the use of child health services. *Pediatrics,* 2007; 119(1): e86-92.
[5] Haun J. N., Patel N. R., French D. D., Campbell R. R., Bradham D. D., Lapcevic W. A. Association between health literacy and medical care costs in an integrated healthcare system: a regional population based study. *BMC Health Serv. Res.,* 2015; 15:249.
[6] Friedland R. New estimates of the high costs of inadequate health literacy. Promoting Health Literacy: A Call to Action; 1998; Washington, D.C.
[7] Vernon J. T. A., Rosenbaum S., DeBuono B. *Low Health Literacy: Implications for National Health Policy.* Storrs, CT: National Bureau of Economic Research (NBER); 2007.
[8] Agarwal N., Shah K., Stone J. G., Ricks C. B., Friedlander R. M. Educational Resources "Over the Head" of Neurosurgical Patients: The Economic Impact of Inadequate Health Literacy. *World Neurosurg,* 2015; 84(5):1223-1226.
[9] Eichler K., Wieser S., Brugger U. The costs of limited health literacy: a systematic review. *Int. J. Public Health,* 2009; 54(5):313-324.
[10] Kutner M., Greenberg, E., Jin, Y., and Paulsen, C. *The Health Literacy of America's Adults: Results From the 2003 National Assessment of Adult Literac.* Washington, D.C.: U.S. Department of Education; 2006.
[11] Paasche-Orlow M. K., Parker R. M., Gazmararian J. A., Nielsen-Bohlman L. T., Rudd RR. The prevalence of limited health literacy. *J. Gen. Intern. Med.,* 2005; 20(2):175-184.
[12] Lantz P. M., House J. S., Lepkowski J. M., Williams D. R., Mero R. P., Chen J. Socioeconomic factors, health behaviors, and mortality: results from a nationally representative prospective study of US adults. *JAMA,* 1998; 279(21):1703-1708.
[13] Marmot M. The influence of income on health: views of an epidemiologist. *Health Aff (Millwood),* 2002; 21(2):31-46.
[14] Sorlie P. D., Backlund E., Keller J. B. US mortality by economic, demographic, and social characteristics: the National Longitudinal Mortality Study. *Am. J. Public Health,* 1995; 85(7):949-956.
[15] Winkleby M. A., Jatulis D. E., Frank E., Fortmann S. P. Socioeconomic status and health: how education, income, and occupation contribute to

risk factors for cardiovascular disease. *Am. J. Public Health,* 1992; 82(6):816-820.

[16] Winkleby M. A., Fortmann S. P., Barrett D. C. Social class disparities in risk factors for disease: eight-year prevalence patterns by level of education. *Prev. Med.,* 1990; 19(1):1-12.

[17] Sanders L. M., Federico S., Klass P., Abrams M. A., Dreyer B. Literacy and child health: a systematic review. *Arch. Pediatr. Adolesc. Med.,* 2009; 163(2):131-140.

[18] Schillinger D., Barton L. R., Karter A. J., Wang F., Adler N. Does literacy mediate the relationship between education and health outcomes? A study of a low-income population with diabetes. *Public Health Rep.,* 2006; 121(3):245-254.

[19] Mottus R., Johnson W., Murray C., Wolf M. S., Starr J. M., Deary I. J. Towards understanding the links between health literacy and physical health. *Health Psychol.,* 2014; 33(2):164-173.

[20] Nutbeam D. Defining and measuring health literacy: what can we learn from literacy studies? *Int. J. Public Health,* 2009; 54(5):303-305.

[21] Waite K. R., Federman A. D., McCarthy D. M., et al. Literacy and race as risk factors for low rates of advance directives in older adults. *J. Am. Geriatr. Soc.,* 2013; 61(3):403-406.

[22] Wolf M. S., Davis T. C., Osborn C. Y., Skripkauskas S., Bennett C. L., Makoul G. Literacy, self-efficacy, and HIV medication adherence. *Patient Educ. Couns.,* 2007; 65(2):253-260.

[23] Heisler M., Bouknight R. R., Hayward R. A., Smith D. M., Kerr E. A. The relative importance of physician communication, participatory decision making, and patient understanding in diabetes self-management. *J. Gen. Intern. Med.,* 2002; 17(4):243-252.

[24] Schillinger D., Piette J., Grumbach K., et al. Closing the loop: physician communication with diabetic patients who have low health literacy. *Arch. Intern. Med.,* 2003; 163(1):83-90.

[25] Keller D. L., Wright J., Pace H. A. Impact of health literacy on health outcomes in ambulatory care patients: a systematic review. *Ann. Pharmacother.,* 2008; 42(9):1272-1281.

[26] Zhang N. J., Terry A., McHorney C. A. Impact of health literacy on medication adherence: a systematic review and meta-analysis. *Ann. Pharmacother.,* 2014; 48(6):741-751.

[27] Osborn C. Y., Paasche-Orlow M. K., Davis T. C., Wolf M. S. Health literacy: an overlooked factor in understanding HIV health disparities. *Am. J. Prev. Med.,* 2007; 33(5):374-378.

[28] Koh H. K., Rudd R. E. The Arc of Health Literacy. *JAMA,* 2015; 314(12):1225-1226.

[29] Schulz P. J., Nakamoto K. Health literacy and patient empowerment in health communication: the importance of separating conjoined twins. *Patient Educ. Couns.,* 2013; 90(1):4-11.

[30] Mackert M., Champlin S., Su Z., Guadagno M. The Many Health Literacies: Advancing Research or Fragmentation? *Health Commun.,* 2015; 30(12):1161-1165.

In: The Evolution of Health Literacy
Editors: N. Agarwal et al.
ISBN: 978-1-53610-602-2

Chapter 7

ASSESSING HEALTH LITERACY IN THE HISPANIC COMMUNITY

Ahmed Jorge, PhD[1], James Zhou[1] and Diego Chaves-Gnecco, MD, MPH[2]
[1]University of Pittsburgh School of Medicine, Pittsburgh, PA, US
[2]Children's Hospital of Pittsburgh, University of Pittsburgh Medical Center, Pittsburgh, PA, US

ABSTRACT

In the United States, the health literacy levels of Spanish-speaking patients exist on a spectrum influenced by the varying degrees of bilingualism and cultural integration observed within this population. Multiple studies have confirmed that the health outcomes of this group are a direct reflection of their health literacy levels. This dynamic association warrants further research with a particular focus on the unique sociolinguistic and socioeconomic characteristics of this population. This chapter explores this topic with special emphasis on clarifying the interactions between language proficiency and health literacy. It then discusses some of the pitfalls that can arise while assessing the health literacy level of a patient from this group. Finally, it provides specific examples of methods to improve health literacy that have been studied and implemented with success in this particular population. The observations and recommendations outlined within this chapter can serve, with appropriate adjustments, as building blocks for similar discussions regarding other bilingual populations within the United States.

The Continuum of Bilingualism in Healthcare

Background

A large number of studies attempting to assess health literacy levels among Hispanics living in the United States have identified several concerning gaps within this population. The National Assessment of Adult Literacy (NAAL), for example, reported low levels of health literacy among the overall Hispanic population in the United States, specifically in men older than 65 years of age [1]. On the other hand, while regional studies have found a direct correlation between education, health literacy and health outcomes, no relationship was observed between gender or age and the aforementioned variables [2, 3]. The aforementioned studies have been limited, however, by several inconsistencies. The NAAL study was performed in 2003, more than a decade ago, and was not designed to account for confounding factors such as varying levels of English proficiency among US Hispanics. Despite these limitations, this study is still widely cited in the literature as one of the few that have tackled the topic of health literacy within the US Hispanic population on a national level [2]. In contrast, some of the studies that have focused on a specific US geographic region have been able to properly address the issue of inconsistent English proficiency, but have failed at conceptualizing the data on a national level. Many of these geographically constrained studies cite high levels of health literacy among the Hispanic population, but their target populations are composed of communities found on the US-Mexico border or communities with high densities of Hispanic healthcare providers, where language is not necessarily a barrier [2, 4-6]. By focusing on specific settings or special zones, these studies may have produced biased results that are not necessarily applicable to the general Hispanic population.

On the whole, prior literature points to variables such as age, educational background and language as the primary determinants of health literacy. However, only a few studies have investigated how these factors influence health literacy in the US Hispanic population specifically [2, 7]. Similarly, the role of bilingualism as a determinant of health literacy has also been understudied. These variables add complexity when attempting to measure health literacy levels in this population. Some of the issues that are explored in this chapter revolve around this notion. For example, how do patients who are well educated in their native language, but possess a limited knowledge of English, compare with patients who have higher English proficiency but lower educational levels? How do Hispanic patients from intertwined communities of expatriates compare to Hispanic patients who have fully integrated in their non-Hispanic communities? These questions delve into the role that acculturation plays in determining the health literacy of US immigrants, and will be further explored in this chapter.

The lack of accurate data and corresponding studies to assess health literacy in US Hispanics is concerning because this population accounts for 16.3% of the US population, or about 50 million people, according to the 2010 US Census [8]. Moreover, the Hispanic population was responsible for most of the total US population growth, or about 56%, from the year 2000 to 2010 [9]. Some regions in the US have even higher densities of Hispanic patients than baseline; for example, in Miami-Dade County and Los Angeles County, 72% and 40% of residents identify Spanish as a language spoken at home, respectively. Given this context, it is understandable why the generally low levels of English proficiency exhibited by this group, compounded with overall low health literacy levels, can produce catastrophic effects for the nation as a whole. For example, this population has an inherently increased risk for developing type 2 diabetes mellitus and non-alcoholic fatty liver disease due to the strong role of population-specific polymorphisms [10-13]. These risk factors, when combined with low health literacy levels, may lead to otherwise preventable poor outcomes.

For the purposes of this discussion, the term Hispanic will encompass people from Spain and Spanish-speaking Latin Americans, but not necessarily those that speak Spanish at any specific level [14]. We will not delve into the discussion of the definition of being Hispanic and how that definition differs from the term Latino. It is important to recognize that, as some experts express, arguments about this terminology can have negative connotations and ramifications in the legal and social realms, and can certainly have an impact on the healthcare of these particular groups [15]. However, the disagreement about terminology does serve as useful a point to begin a discussion about the intrinsic heterogeneity of the US Hispanic population, which is the focus of the following section.

The Intrinsic Heterogeneity of the US Hispanic Population

The established healthcare organizational scheme in the United States is a complex nonlinear system with a multitude of variables. As discussed in previous chapters, in this system a patient's comprehension of their illness and relevant medical care is directly correlated with his or her health literacy. The addition of a heterogeneous group of patients, such as bilingual population with varying levels of English proficiency, undoubtedly adds another layer of complexity to the system. It is reasonable to assume, as is the case every day in many hospitals across the nation, that one of the characteristics of such a system is its ability to self-adapt with different patient populations. This ability to self-adapt, however, does not necessarily imply that the results from varying patient populations will replicate the desired goals of care [16]. Furthermore, when attempting to identify and address health literacy concerns, the same strategies discussed in earlier chapters may not be the optimal solution for patients from the Hispanic population. The following section of this chapter discusses the intricacies that play a role in identifying and addressing health literacy concerns when dealing with this particular population.

When considering the US Hispanic population on a more detailed level, the aforementioned "layer of complexity" further fragments into innumerable sub-layers that exponentially add to the discussion of population heterogeneity. The Hispanic population in the United States, while unified by some commonalities such as a common background language, is composed of people from multiple races, ethnicities, nationalities, and cultural backgrounds. Moreover, many people in the US that self-identify as Hispanic do not necessarily speak Spanish at any level. This multitude of variables plays a significant role in influencing the ability of US Hispanics to understanding health and disease.

In addition to these patient-level variables, environmental variables such as the city where an immigrant has settled may also affect how they interact with the healthcare system. Many immigrants are firmly rooted to a complex communal network of family, friends, and neighbors who interact with each other and may add to or subtract from their communal health literacy. For instance, immigrants with a dynamic network of friends and family who speak their native language and possess similar cultural backgrounds are able to circumnavigate language barriers without addressing their deficiencies in the language of their host country [2]. Other immigrants settle in communities where they are immersed almost completely by their host country's language culture, effectively falling into the dominion of the health literacy issues discussed in previous chapters.

It is important to recall that the heterogeneity that exists within the US Hispanic population, especially in regards to health literacy, must also be viewed in the context of our discussions in previous chapters. Members of the Hispanic subset of the US population experience the same health literacy issues as their native counterparts. They are still required to make decisions about their healthcare regardless of where they may fall in the continuum of health literacy. For example, this population will use modern technology to assess and complement their health education in the same manner as non-Hispanic US residents. Because of this, healthcare providers must endeavor to treat this population with the same vigilance that they utilize for other populations with limited health literacy.

In summary, the US Hispanic population, along with many other bilingual groups in the United States, is a highly heterogeneous entity defined by multiple variables such varying levels of bilingualism, inconsistent integration into US culture, and different underlying levels of health literacy. Recognition of this fact is important for all healthcare providers because any foundation of health literacy will be built upon each patient's individual background. The next section will discuss how the heterogeneity within the US Hispanic population affects the way in which members of this population interact with and benefit from the American healthcare system.

How Heterogeneity within the US Hispanic Population Affects the Healthcare System

The spectrum of backgrounds observed in US Hispanics can more easily conceptualized for the healthcare professional by defining three main pillars of heterogeneity: language differences, health literacy differences, and cultural differences. By keeping these three pillars in mind, the health care provider is able to assess the baseline health literacy of this group with clearer understanding and better judgment [16]. It is important to recognize that while these three basic pillars form the foundation for an approach to this population, they are not exhaustive.

The first pillar, language differences, delves into how the lack of a common language can be a barrier for the patient-provider (health provider) relationship. With over 8% of the population self-identifying as limited English proficiency, this is a major concern for the healthcare field [8]. For example, some physicians may attempt to overcome a perceived language barrier with the use of non-verbal communications. However, the use of non-verbal communications sets the tone of a clinic visit to an elementary level, and precludes the necessary communication necessary to accomplish the goals of routine patient care.

Many clinicians will also encounter barriers when attempting to verbally communicate with non-English speaking patients. Not only will patients often overestimate their English proficiency, but physicians and other healthcare providers may also overestimate their knowledge of medical Spanish [7]. A physician's inability to correctly identify a patient's inherent level of English proficiency, or a physician overestimating his/her ability to communicate in medical Spanish may set the stage for misunderstanding and confusion during patient-clinician interactions.

The ability to correctly assess the English proficiency of a US Hispanic patient is crucial; studies have shown that one of most important predictors of health literacy is English proficiency [2]. On the same note, it is also important for healthcare professionals to their own knowledge of Spanish in order to prevent inadvertent miscommunication, however well-intentioned. One study revealed that 21 out of 40 of health professionals at a pediatric institution use Spanish to communicate diagnostic evaluations, medication regimens, and discharge instructions to patients, even though they considered their Spanish level to be "non-proficient" [17]. Another study revealed that in a pediatric setting, 53% of interpreter errors had significant clinical consequences. In one particular case, a combination of interpreter errors, in both the language and cultural domains lead to a male infant being discharged with life-threatening medical conditions [18].

In light of the previous discussion, physicians must also exercise care when using a commercially or publically available test to categorize a bilingual patient's language proficiency. Many of the tools found in the literature designed to assess the health literacy level among Spanish speakers vary widely in how, and in what context, they measure health literacy [19]. These tools require that the savvy health practitioner investigate further into other intricacies besides language differences that may affect each patient's intrinsic health literacy level. Factors other than raw English language proficiency, such as a patient's intrinsic health literacy level in his/her native tongue, should also be taken into account when planning how to communicate with a US Hispanic patient [2].

The second pillar of heterogeneity consists of the underlying differences in baseline health literacy observed within the US Hispanic population. A study highlighting differences in the care of the Hispanic immigrant population in Boston versus the Hispanic immigrant population in Spain (where Spanish is the national language) demonstrates the importance of health literacy differences after normalizing for language differences. Among other factors, a low health literacy level correlated with lower service utilization regardless of location. Other barriers, such as non-familiarity with treatment options and difficulty navigating to healthcare locations, were cited in this study as significant impediments to care regardless of whether patients resided in the US or in Spain [20]. These findings highlight the importance of baseline health literacy in all patients, including Hispanics. They also demonstrate how, even with a common language, immigrants can encounter attitudinal and structural barriers that limit their interactions with their healthcare providers.

The final pillar of heterogeneity comprises the cultural differences intrinsic to the US Hispanic population. As described in the previous section, even within the same country of origin, cultural characteristics within an individual group can vary immensely. Each individual immigrant will invariably adopt some beliefs and practices of the host culture while simultaneously discarding part of their native background, a process defined as acculturation [21]. The degree to which an immigrant adopts the culture of his/her host country can either benefit or detract from his/her healthcare outcomes. In many instances, this process of complex exchanges has been associated with negative effects on the healthcare of immigrants. Many aspects of adapting to a new setting, such as adopting new dietary customs, following new exercise routines, and developing a heavier dependence on electronic health media, can have profound effects on healthcare outcomes in the immigrant population. One study revealed that an e-Health weight loss tool previously found to be effective in native US residents required additional adjustments in order to retain effectiveness in an immigrant population due to cultural, dietary, and language-related idiosyncrasies within that group [22].

On the topic of acculturation, previous studies have suggested that an immigrant's degree of acculturation can influence healthcare outcomes as much as country of origin. For instance, Puerto Rican populations with higher levels of acculturation were found to have higher rates of major cardiovascular disease risk factors when compared to similar populations with lower levels of acculturation [23, 24]. Other studies also suggest that an immigrant's degree of acculturation can influence healthcare as strongly as birthplace. Higher rates of gastric cancer were found in Hispanic men from a variety of nationalities, ranging from Mexicans to Puerto Ricans and Cubans, corresponding to higher levels of acculturation independent of nationality [25]. First- or second-generation Hispanic men, but interestingly not Hispanic women, were found to have a higher prevalence of obesity when compared to foreign born Hispanic men [26]. Low levels of acculturation have also been associated with worsened health outcomes for US Hispanics. Newly immigrated Hispanics (a surrogate variable for acculturation) in San Francisco were found to have a higher incidence of *H. pylori* infection [27]. In a Chicago Hispanic population-based study, a lower level of acculturation was found to be associated with higher rates of breast cancer due to delays in seeking diagnosis and treatment [28]. In groups of Hispanics and Native Americans in Kansas, low acculturation levels have also been found to be a major factor in the ability to afford the Papanicolaou test, a regular diagnostic tool used in the detection of cervical cancer [29].

Conversely, certain types of acculturation may have a positive impact on the healthcare outcomes observed in immigrant groups. A longer time spent in the host country can improve outcomes by providing increasing access to healthcare, health insurance, and preventive health services [30].

It is important to understand that a majority of the preceding studies have been limited by a number of constraints due to their focus on specific sub-regions within the United States. By virtue of their design, these studies focus on very specific populations, each defined by differing parameters and comprising their own individual heterogeneous spectrums. Because of the disparity between the populations studied by these papers, there are contradictions as to how much of an effect acculturation has on healthcare outcomes. A recent systematic review revealed that a US-born Hispanics and Hispanic immigrants with more than 10 years in the country were consuming significantly more sugar or sugar-sweetened beverages than their less-acculturated immigrant counterparts. However, at the same time, this review concluded that the level of acculturation was not associated with dietary intake of cholesterol, and that evidence to support an association between acculturation and fruit and fiber intake was mixed [31]. Many of the disparities reported in this study can be attributed to the issues previously discussed; namely, a narrow geographical boundary, a lack of distinct Hispanic subgroups, and a lack of analysis over time.

Furthermore, some researchers argue that acculturation is not the most appropriate variable when assessing the Hispanic population when developing a comprehensive health literacy library. Their argument is that other factors such as social and economic inequalities and discrimination play a much more relevant role than acculturation itself [32]. Some even consider the term acculturation as a “catch-all construct” that dangerously circumnavigates the preceding issues [33, 34]. One aspect of these arguments fixates on the idea of focusing on specific ethnic particularities of this group with a careful look at cultural context, instead of delving further into the inconsistent notion of acculturation [35].

Once more, it is important to keep in mind that US Hispanics are also affect by the general health literacy issues described in previous chapters. For example, preventive care utilization such as influenza and pneumococcal vaccination and mammograms is lower in low health literacy groups regardless of ethnic background or acculturation levels [36]. Additionally, inefficient resource use can result in thousands of dollars of unnecessary costs when caring for patients with inadequate health literacy, regardless of whether these patients are Hispanic or native US residents [37].

This section served to outline the multitude of factors that affect how US Hispanic patients interact with the healthcare system, and the ways in which those factors affect patient outcomes in this particular population. The preceding discussion facilitated the focus of this chapter by creating three conceptual pillars of the heterogeneity within the US Hispanic. Even after simplifying the group into these three dimensions, we demonstrate that the foundation of the health literacy in this group is complex and should be tackled at a personal level. In the next sections, we explore some aspects of assessing the bilingual patients from the point of view of the healthcare provider. We also delve into some tasks that are heavily influenced by the ethnicity, language fluency, cultural origin, and health literacy of each individual patient.

ASSESSING THE BILINGUAL PATIENT

Evaluating Decision Making Capacity in the Bilingual Patient

The communication goals of the medical team should reach beyond simply establishing an elementary form of health literacy in a patient. The goal of communication should be to explore the perspective of the patient, understand his/her point of view, and elicit his/her expectations and goals for healthcare. In turn, such communication forms the foundation of the patient's care in regards to assessing their decision-making capacity and obtaining informed consent.

Factors that should be in the mind of the healthcare professional when assessing the need to engage the bilingual patient include distinguishing between different clinical situations, the availability of resources, the degree of English proficiency (addressed previously) and each patient's individual preferences [38]. Different clinical situations will inevitably change what tools a health professional selects to best communicate with a patient.

One of these tools, the use of an interpreter, has been correlated with higher patient satisfaction and better healthcare outcomes, undoubtedly improving the patient-provider relationship and ultimately founding a building block towards improving the patient's health literacy status [39]. Nonetheless, some have identified an alarming underuse of this tool by health professionals despite the knowledge of the aforementioned benefits. Many healthcare providers report being constrained for time, others believe hand gestures are sufficient, and still others are unaware of the availability of such resources at their institution [40]. Neglecting to utilize such resources during certain scenarios may worsen healthcare outcomes. A note of caution: physicians must exercise care when attempting to overcome the lack of an official interpreter by utilizing family members as unofficial interpreters. Many have proposed prohibiting children younger than 15 years of age from serving as interpreters due to their inherent lack of competency in medical terminology and documented risks for significant medical mistakes [41].

The availability of resources differs based on institution. However, some commonalities exist. Legal entities have established significant precedent regarding discrimination against an individual based on his/her language, and have thus created minimum standards to be acknowledged by every health care institution, especially when government funds are utilized [42-44]. Because of these mandates, each medical institution must maintain adequate access to interpreter resources, while also balancing the cost such resources represent to the institution. For instance, while an in-house trained interpreter is obviously the optimal solution, many institutions may resort to suboptimal solutions such as telephone interpreters that may unnecessarily delay communications and ultimately treatment [39].

Understanding Health Literacy in the Context of Cultural Competency

Cultural competency in the field of medicine is challenging for any health professional. While it is unfeasible for all healthcare professionals to be fluent in every culture that may be encountered, there are core cross-cultural issues that all such professionals should be familiar with. Moreover, practitioners should acquire the ability to assess and act according to a common set of principles based on different cultural beliefs, language preferences, values and attitudes even if an on-site interpreter is available.

Although there are challenging issues that transcend ethnicity and race, certain themes are more common in the Hispanic population. For example, a study revealed that in a population of patients in Los Angeles, a patients that self-identified as Hispanic were much more likely to prefer family-centered environments, rather than the typical model of autonomy found in the US [45] Similarly, a study revealed that Hispanic healthcare practitioners are uncomfortable with the US practice of discussing all healthcare information directly with each patient, especially in cases dealing with terminal diagnoses [46].

IMPROVING HEALTH LITERACY IN THE HISPANIC POPULATION

In the previous sections we discussed the intrinsic heterogeneity of the US Hispanic population, and how that heterogeneity affects each patient's individual level of health literacy. This section outlines a list of specific tools, which although not exhaustive in nature, can be used as a first step to facilitate interactions with patients in this specific group. These tools should be used while keeping in mind each patient's individuals needs and understanding that those needs may evolve as the patient's situation changes. Moreover, the healthcare professional should be aware of his or her own limitations in assessing the degree to which the patient's background affects his/her health literacy. Understanding and assessing one's own level in a language is the first step when using any of the following tools.

The following examples make use of culturally attuned values, relevant metaphors and proverbs, and imaginative visual aids to tailor healthcare communication to members of this population. Nonetheless, special care must be exercised when deciding which tools to utilize based on an individual patient's characteristics. For example, it is important to realize that a well-educated patient with a higher health literacy level but low English proficiency might not be as interested in visually diluted content as another patient with a lower health literacy level.

Novel Tools Used in Specific Settings

Disparities in health literacy and healthcare outcomes vary according to factors such as language, race, ethnicity, and income level. Simple interventions are able to mitigate these disparities. In the case of a colorectal cancer (CRC) screening effectiveness randomized clinical trial, a simple modification to the pre-existing standard of care was able to increase adherence in a patient pool composed of 87% Hispanics with the majority uninsured. The low cost intervention consisted of a mailed reminder letter and a screening kit with specific instructions tailored to the patient's level of education [47]. The trial reported an outstanding 82% rate of compliance, which arguably improved the care of all patients involved.

In the pediatric emergency room setting, a kiosk was implemented to triage bilingual patients with non-urgent conditions. The kiosk consisted of a multi touch computer screen that collected information regarding the chief complaint and relevant medical history. In this randomized clinical trial, time to complete triage was significantly shorter and inaccuracies were significantly lower for the kiosk group when compared to the standard nurse group [48]. Thus, this implementation was able to elegantly resolve many of the issues outlined in our previous discussion. For example, the automated computer system was able to quickly translate a constellation of symptoms and complaints to the health professional while minimizing misunderstandings, indisputably an important aspect of emergency medical care. In the future, a kiosk of this type may be able to identify specific subgroups and target pertinent patient-tailored educational material to improve health literacy after every single visit.

Use of a Fotonovela

Multiple clinical trials across many disciplines in medicine have evaluated the use of the fotonovela to improve health literacy in the Hispanic community. A fotonovela, or a picture book with captions, usually depicts a dramatic story where actors showcase their experiences navigating particular aspects of their health. This tool fuses the areas of patient education and entertainment, with the ultimate goal being to incorporate important health literacy content into popular culture. The premise is to engage the audience with a familiar form of entertainment, thus helping them internalize the health concern and motivating them to discover and contemplate their options. In addition, these fotonovelas are grounded in evidence-based medicine and are custom-made to address specific cultural misperceptions. Some of these studies pay particular attention to details, such as performing a preliminary study regarding current attitudes towards the particular disease, in order to form the content of the fotonovela. Moreover, the team working on the fotonovela is typically composed of healthcare professionals that ground the storyline with evidence based medicine and cultural appropriate content.

One randomized clinical trial assessed the effect of a bilingual fotonovela on the attitudes, knowledge, and behavior in Hispanic adults in Los Angeles suffering from depression. The fotonovela in this trial focused on addressing common misconceptions regarding the diagnosis and treatment of depression in these particular communities. Common but complex issues that were explored included topics such as the degree to which psychotropic medications can alleviate the symptoms of depression, the potential for addiction to such medications, and the necessary duration of psychotropic therapy. The study concluded that the mental health stigma associated with depression was markedly reduced in the group assigned to the fotonovela when compared to the group assigned to a standard bilingual text pamphlet. Moreover, the knowledge retained during a one-month follow up was also significantly greater in the fotonovela group [49].

CONCLUSION

In this chapter, we have explored a number of topics relevant to the healthcare literacy of Hispanic patients in the United States. First, we demonstrated that the term "Hispanic" comprises a population with a high degree of intrinsic heterogeneity. We then simplified the heterogeneity of this population in regards to the healthcare system by establishing three conceptual pillars: language differences, cultural differences, and baseline healthcare literacy differences. We provided specific examples of each pillar, and in so doing outlined a basic approach for physicians to interact with US Hispanic and other bilingual patients. Finally, we provided specific examples of tools and systems used in prior studies that have shown promise in improving the relationship between physicians and Hispanic patients, and thus improving healthcare outcomes in this group. The content of this chapter may serve as a blueprint for similar interactions with other bilingual immigrants groups within the United States.

REFERENCES

[1] US Department of Education. National Assessment of Adult Literacy (NAAL): A First Look at the Literacy of America's Adults in the 21st Century. In: *Sciences IoE*, ed. Vol. NCES Publication No. 2006-470. Washington, D.C. 2006.

[2] Jacobson HE, Hund L, Soto-Mas F. Predictors of English Health Literacy among US Hispanic Immigrants: The importance of language, bilingualism and sociolinguistic environment. *Literacy and numeracy studies: an international journal in the education and training of adults.* 2016;24(1):43-64.

[3] Boyas JF. Correlates of health literacy among latinos in Arkansas. *Soc. Work Public Health.* 2013;28(1).

[4] Penaranda E, Diaz M, Noriega O, Shokar N. Evaluation of Health Literacy among Spanish-Speaking Primary Care Patients Along the US-Mexico Border. *Public Health and Environmental Medicine.* 2012;105 (7).

[5] Soto-Mas F, Mein E, Fuentes B, Thatcher B, Balcazar H. Integrating health literacy and ESL: an interdisciplinary curriculum for Hispanic immigrants. *Health promotion practice.* Mar. 2013;14(2):263-273.

[6] Ko E, Zuniga ML, Peacher D, Palomino H, Watson M. Efficacy of Cancer Care Communication Between Clinicians and Latino Patients in a Rural US-Mexico Border Region: a Qualitative Study of Barriers and Facilitators to Better Communication. *Journal of cancer education: the official journal of the American Association for Cancer Education.* Aug. 25 2016.

[7] Wilson-Stronks A, Galvez E. *Hospitals, Language, and Culture: A Snapshot of the Nation.* Oakbrook Terrace, IL: The Joint Commission; 2007.

[8] US Census Bureau, State and County QuickFacts. 2013. Accessed August, 2016.

[9] Passel J, Cohn D, Lopez M. Hispanics Account for More Than Half of Nation's Growth in Past Decade. *Pew Research Center Hispanic Trends.* 2011.

[10] Piccolo RS, Subramanian SV, Pearce N, Florez JC, McKinlay JB. Relative Contributions of Socioeconomic, Local Environmental, Psychosocial, Lifestyle/Behavioral, Biophysiological, and Ancestral Factors to Racial/Ethnic Disparities in Type 2 Diabetes. *Diabetes Care.* 2016;1208(17).

[11] Lazo M, Bilal U, Perez-Escamilla R. Epidemiology of NAFLD and Type 2 Diabetes: Health Disparities Among Persons of Hispanic Origin. *Current diabetes reports.* Dec. 2015;15(12):116.

[12] Lewis EF, Claggett B, Parfrey PS et al. Race and ethnicity influences on cardiovascular and renal events in patients with diabetes mellitus. *American heart journal.* Aug. 2015; 170(2):322-329.

[13] Duggan C, Carosso E, Mariscal N, Islas I. *Diabetes Prevention in Hispanics: Report From a Randomized Controlled Trial.* Centers for Disease Control and Prevention; 2014.

[14] Revisions to the Standards for the Classification of Federal Data on Race and Ethnicity. Federal Register Notice. *Office of Management and Budget* 1997. Accessed August 29, 2016, 2016.

[15] Taylor D, Morales JV. *Negotiating performance: gender, sexuality, and theatricality in Latin/o America.* Duke University Press; 1994.

[16] Schyve PM. Language differences as a barrier to quality and safety in health care: the Joint Commission perspective. *Journal of general internal medicine.* Nov. 2007;22 Suppl. 2:360-361.

[17] Sonja C, O'Leary B, Federico S, Hampers L. The Truth About Language Barriers: One Residency Program's Experience. *Pediatrics* 2003;111(5).

[18] Flores G, Abreu M, Schwartz I, Hill M. The importance of language and culture in pediatric care: case studies from the Latino community. *The Journal of pediatrics.* Dec. 2000;137(6):842-848.

[19] Stonbraker S, Schnall R, Larson E. Tools to measure health literacy among Spanish speakers: An integrative review of the literature. *Patient education and counseling.* Jul. 21 2015.

[20] Falgas I, Ramos Z, Herrera L et al. Barriers to and Correlates of Retention in Behavioral Health Treatment Among Latinos in 2 Different Host Countries: The United States and Spain. *Journal of public health management and practice: JPHMP.* Feb. 23 2016.

[21] Zambrana RE, Carter-Pokras O. Role of acculturation research in advancing science and practice in reducing health care disparities among Latinos. *Am. J. Public Health.* 2010;18(23).

[22] Steven S. Coughlin DH, and Lee S. Caplan. The need for culturally-tailored smartphone applications for weight control. *J. Ga Public Health Assoc.* 2016;5(3).

[23] Daviglus ML, Talavera GA, Aviles-Santa ML et al. Prevalence of major cardiovascular risk factors and cardiovascular diseases among Hispanic/Latino individuals of diverse backgrounds in the United States. *Jama.* Nov. 7 2012;308(17):1775-1784.

[24] Gallo LC, Roesch SC, Fortmann AL et al. Associations of chronic stress burden, perceived stress, and traumatic stress with cardiovascular disease prevalence and risk factors in the Hispanic Community Health Study/Study of Latinos Sociocultural Ancillary Study. *Psychosomatic medicine.* Jul-Aug. 2014;76(6):468-475.

[25] Chang ET, Gomez SL, Fish K et al. Gastric cancer incidence among Hispanics in California: patterns by time, nativity, and neighborhood characteristics. *Cancer epidemiology, biomarkers and prevention: a publication of the American Association for Cancer Research, cosponsored by the American Society of Preventive Oncology.* May 2012;21(5):709-719.

[26] *UCLA Center for Health Policy Research, California Department of Health Services, Public Health Institute.* 2001-2011.

[27] Tsai CJ, Perry S, Sanchez L, Parsonnet J. Helicobacter pylori infection in different generations of Hispanics in the San Francisco Bay Area. *American journal of epidemiology.* Aug. 15 2005;162(4):351-357.

[28] Tejeda S, Gallardo RI, Ferrans CE, Rauscher GH. Breast cancer delay in Latinas: the role of cultural beliefs and acculturation. *Journal of behavioral medicine.* Aug. 29 2016.

[29] Moreland S, Engelman K, Greiner K, Mayo MS. Papanicolaou testing among Native American and Hispanic populations. *Ethn. Dis.* 2006;16 (1).

[30] Lopez L, Grant RW, Marceau L, Piccolo R, McKinlay JB, Meigs JB. Association of Acculturation and Health Literacy with Prevalent Dysglycemia and Diabetes Control Among Latinos in the Boston Area Community Health (BACH) Survey. *Journal of immigrant and minority health/Center for Minority Public Health.* Feb. 22 2016.

[31] Ayala GX, Baquero B, Klinger S. A systematic review of the relationship between acculturation and diet among Latinos in the United States: implications for future research. *Journal of the American Dietetic Association.* Aug. 2008;108(8):1330-1344.

[32] Viruell-Fuentes EA. Beyond acculturation: immigration, discrimination, and health research among Mexicans in the United States. *Social science and medicine.* Oct. 2007; 65(7):1524-1535.

[33] James SA. Racial and ethnic differences in infant mortality and low birth weight. A psychosocial critique. *Annals of Epidemiology.* 1993;3(2).

[34] Adrados R. Drug abuse among minority youth: Advances in research and methodology. In: De La Rosa J-LRA, ed. *Acculturation: The*

broader view. Theoretical framework of acculturation scales. Rockville, MD: National Institute of Drug Abuse; 1993.

[35] Hunt LM, Schneider S, Comer B. Should "acculturation" be a variable in health research? A critical review of research on US Hispanics. *Social science and medicine.* Sep. 2004;59(5):973-986.

[36] Scott T, Gazmararian J, Williams BA, Baker DW. Health Literacy and Preventive Health Care Use Among Medicare Enrollees in a Managed Care Organization. *Medical Care.* 2002;40(5).

[37] Howard DH, Gazmararian J, Parker RM. The impact of low health literacy on the medical costs of Medicare managed care enrollees. *The American journal of medicine.* Apr. 2005;118(4):371-377.

[38] Yael Schenker MBL, MD; Katharine M. Ettinger, JD; and Alicia Fernandez, MD. Navigating Language Barriers under Difficult Circumstances. *Annals of Internal Medicine.* 2008;149.

[39] Dueweke AR, Bridges AJ, Gomez DP. The Effects of Interpreter Use on Agreement Between Clinician- and Self-Ratings of Functioning in Hispanic Integrated Care Patients. *Journal of immigrant and minority health/Center for Minority Public Health.* Sep. 29 2015.

[40] Diamond LC, Schenker Y, Curry L, Bradley EH, Fernandez A. Getting by: underuse of interpreters by resident physicians. *Journal of general internal medicine.* Feb. 2009;24 (2):256-262.

[41] Flores G. Language Barriers to Health Care in the United States. *N. Engl. J. Med.* 2006; 355(3).

[42] Chen AH, Youdelman MK, Brooks J. The legal framework for language access in healthcare settings: Title VI and beyond. *Journal of general internal medicine.* Nov. 2007;22 Suppl. 2:362-367.

[43] Perkins J, Youdelman M, Wong D. *Ensuring Linguistic Access in Health Care Settings: Legal Rights And Responsibilities.* 2nd ed. Washington, DC: National Health Law Program; 2003.

[44] Grubbs V, Chen A, Bindman A, Vittinghoff E, Fernandez A. Effect of awareness of language law on language access in the health care setting. *Journal of general internal medicine.* 2006;21(7).

[45] Blackhall L, Murphy S, Frank G, Michel V, Azen S. Ethnicity and attitudes toward patient autonomy. *Jama.* 1995;274(10):820.

[46] Braun UK, Ford ME, Beyth RJ, McCullough LB. The physician's professional role in end-of-life decision-making: voices of racially and ethnically diverse physicians. *Patient education and counseling.* Jul. 2010;80(1):3-9.

[47] Baker DW, Brown T, Buchanan DR et al. Comparative effectiveness of a multifaceted intervention to improve adherence to annual colorectal cancer screening in community health centers: a randomized clinical trial. *JAMA internal medicine.* Aug. 2014;174(8): 1235-1241.

[48] Sinha M, Khor K, Amresh A, Drachman D, Frechette A. The Use of a Kiosk-Model Bilingual Self-Triage System in the Pediatric Emergency Department. *Pediatric Emergency Care.* 2014;30(1).

[49] Unger JB, Cabassa LJ, Molina GB, Contreras S, Baron M. Evaluation of a fotonovela to increase depression knowledge and reduce stigma among Hispanic adults. *Journal of immigrant and minority health/Center for Minority Public Health.* Apr. 2013;15(2): 398-406.

About the Editors

Nitin Agarwal, M.D.
Neurological Surgery Resident
Department of Neurological Surgery,
University of Pittsburgh Medical Center,
Pittsburgh, Pennsylvania

Nitin Agarwal, MD, matriculated into the University of Pittsburgh Department of Neurological Surgery residency program in 2014. Prior to joining, Dr. Agarwal received his doctorate of medicine from Rutgers New Jersey Medical School. His funded research interests focus on improving patient education to optimize clinical outcomes. To date, he has published over 100 peer-reviewed articles and book chapters as well as spoken at several national conferences with over 75 oral and poster presentations. His health literary related research has been published in several high impact factor journals including *JAMA Internal Medicine* and featured by prominent healthcare oriented news outlets such as *Reuters Health*. Dr. Agarwal also maintains an active role in organized neurosurgery advocating for medical student as well as patient education. Recently, he was appointed as a member of the Young Neurosurgeons Committee of the American Association of Neurological Surgeons and selected as a Council of State Neurological Societies socioeconomic fellow. Outside of medicine, Dr. Agarwal is deeply dedicated to martial arts, specifically the disciplines of Taekwondo, Krav Maga, and Jiu-Jitsu.

David R. Hansberry, M.D., Ph.D.
Radiology Resident
Department of Radiology, Thomas Jefferson University Hospitals,
Philadelphia, Pennsylvania

David Hansberry, MD, PhD, is a radiology resident in Philadelphia, Pennsylvania at Thomas Jefferson University Hospitals. Prior to joining Jefferson, Dr. Hansberry completed an internship in the department of medicine at Drexel University College of Medicine at Hahnemann Hospital. Dr. Hansberry is a graduate of Rutgers New Jersey Medical School. In addition to his medical degree, Dr. Hansberry holds a PhD and MS in biomedical engineering, which he obtained from Drexel University prior to medical school. He is a graduate of Rutgers University's School of Engineering having completed a BS in biomedical engineering with a minor in physical chemistry. Dr. Hansberry has published widely on topics such as patient education and health literacy, clinical medicine, engineering education, translational research as well as basic science. Dr. Hansberry holds patents and has been involved in technology commercialization. Outside of his clinical and academic pursuits, Dr. Hansberry enjoys spending time with his wife, two kids, and yellow Labrador retriever.

Arpan V. Prabhu
University of Pittsburgh School of Medicine,
Pittsburgh, Pennsylvania

Arpan V. Prabhu, B.S., is a strong proponent for improving health literacy and intercultural communication skills to better relationships among doctors and their patients. To date, he has published 30 peer-reviewed publications and has given 28 oral and poster presentations at national and regional conferences. His health literacy-related research has been published in prominent medical journals, including the *International Journal of Radiation Oncology*Biology*Physics and Practical Radiation Oncology*. Over the last decade, he has received educational grants from universities and nonprofit organizations to study and conduct research abroad on intercultural medicine in central Bolivia and various countries across Asia and Africa. Back home in Pittsburgh, Mr. Prabhu practices the principles learned abroad by volunteering at a Spanish health clinic through Pittsburgh's Children's Hospital, providing comfort and assurance to young patients in their native tongue. Mr. Prabhu's humanities interests include medical poetry and the history of medicine; he has published poems reflecting on medical experiences in the *Medical Humanities* journal and has published multiple historical manuscripts on scientists who have made substantial contributions to the advancement of medicine and science. In his free time, Mr. Prabhu enjoys performing long-form improv comedy and playing basketball.

INDEX

D

E

F

G

H

N

O

P